MW01140008

Food Intolerances

Fructose Malabsorption,
Lactose and Histamine Intolerance

living and eating well after diagnosis
& dealing with the elimination diet

A guide and cook book by
Michael Zechmann

In collaboration with Genny Masterman

With over 40 easily digestible recipes

1st Edition 2013 | ISBN-13: 978-1481020312 | ISBN-10: 1481020315

Impress: Michael Zechmann, Innstraße, 6020 Innsbruck, Austria

            office@society-for-public-health.com

All illustrations and texts © Michael Zechmann | Cover: Image © Elenathewise - Fotolia.com
Photo Genny Masterman by Andreas Komenda | Photo of Michael Zechmann by Foto Hofer
Design by **panthera.cc** | Translation by Sue Masterman

CONTENTS

1. FOREWORD

Is healthy eating, such as vegetables, fruit, honey or fruit juices, giving you problems? If you have been diagnosed with fructose intolerance or fructose malabsorption, then fructose – fruit sugar – is the cause. It is not being properly absorbed by your intestine and then passes on to a further part of the digestive tract where it meets up with bacteria which process this sugar. This results in gas, nausea, abdominal cramps and often diarrhoea as well. That's what happened to me too. After years and years of misdiagnosis which ranged from gastritis to mental illness, I was diagnosed with fructose intolerance and lactose intolerance. That was nearly 10 years ago. At the time there was hardly any public information available on this subject. Because I am a biologist and thus had access to scientific literature through the University, I started to do some research. After I had been researching intensively for more than a year I decided it was time to share my knowledge and as a result I founded an awareness campaign and a website for the German language area. This website has meanwhile become the point of contact for tens of thousands of those affected. While I was working on the website I got to know the journalist and author Genny Masterman, who is also affected. We have meanwhile worked together on several projects related to food intolerances.

Both of us know how it feels when you get a diagnosis and then have to face it alone. With no support, no information, and mostly without any further help from the doctor. Dr. Google is often the first point of call but the baffling choice of websites that meanwhile exist are enough to make your head spin. It is often hard to differentiate between the top quality websites and those of lesser value. But that is precisely what is important in the medical field. After all, this is about your health and your quality of life!

That's why we decided to write a book. We published it in 2012 for the German market and because the response was so good, we decided to translate the book into English. In 2013 we did some research in the U.S. and the UK to adapt the book for the English language area. Its main purpose is to help those who have been given the diagnosis of "fructose malabsorption" or "dietary fructose intolerance". But the book is also meant to be an additional aid for all those who have known about their fructose intolerance for longer and it can additionally be a guide for those suffering from lactose and/or histamine intolerance.

With this book, we hope to contribute to your wellbeing and hope that we can explain as well as is possible about the period following the diagnosis and everything you need to know about it. We also recommend that you read other books, browse through websites (with the necessary caution) and look for counselling from a dietician. You are going to have to come to terms with your nutrition in order to get a positive result. But never do this blindly, always think carefully, listen to your body and only do whatever does you good.

Find your personal tolerance level!

Michael Zechmann & Genny Masterman
April 2013

2. INTOLERANCE, ALLERGY OR MALABSORPTION?

Your diagnosis probably reads "fructose malabsorption" (FM) or "dietary fructose intolerance (DFI) or "intestinal fructose intolerance" (IFI). There is also "hereditary fructose intolerance" (HFI; see page 43), but this is a completely different form, extremely rare and would already have been diagnosed when you were a baby. The terms "fructose malabsorption" and "fructose intolerance" are frequently used in the public domain to describe dietary fructose intolerance. For this reason we will also be using this description in this book.

FOOD ALLERGIES

Food allergies are yet again something different. In the case of these allergies, the body's immune system reacts to a certain substance in the food. The result is typical allergy symptoms such as sneezing, a runny nose, rashes, breathlessness or palpitations. In certain circumstances allergies can be life-threatening, whereas food intolerances are normally not.

The number of adults suffering from food allergies is estimated to be around five to seven per cent of the population in continental Europe. The "National Institute of Allergy and Infectious Diseases" reports that approximately 4 per cent of adults in the United States suffer from food allergies. So let's say it's a range of 4 to 7 per cent in the Western world. Food intolerances, on the other hand, are significantly more frequent, with fructose malabsorption occurring in around 30% of the European population. Allergies occur more frequently in children than in adults. They mostly decrease as people get older. Substances that trigger allergies are also different for children compared to adults. The main allergy triggers for children are cows' milk, soy and eggs. Adults react more frequently to raw fruits and vegetables, nuts, peanuts and some spices. In a large-scale survey carried out by our German website we were able to show that those with intolerances suffered more frequently from certain allergies compared to the rest of the population. This, however, involves mainly pollen and house mite allergies. Since these allergies can also show cross-reactions to food allergies, you should also have an allergy test carried out as well as an intolerance test. Better to be sure!

An Intolerance involves substances, often carbohydrates, which cannot be digested properly. This means they cause problems that mostly occur in the intestine. Larger quantities are needed to cause symptoms. Small quantities are often well tolerated.

The difference between Allergy and Intolerance
An Allergy involves the immune system. Minute substances, often proteins, which the body tries to fight with antibodies (immunoglobulins), give rise to a strong reaction. The smallest quantity is sufficient to cause symptoms.

THE DIFFERENCE BETWEEN MALABSORPTION AND INTOLERANCE

Let's first take a look at the concept of "**Maldigestion**". Maldigestion means "poor digestion" – the substance concerned is not sufficiently split up in the stomach or small intestine and cannot thus be properly digested. That is a medical concept that does not go into detail; it is very superficial and is often used when the physiological cause of the symptoms is unclear.

"**Malabsorption**" on the other hand means "poor absorption". The substance concerned can only be absorbed with difficulty or not at all by the digestive system and thus by the body itself. Here, the physiological factor is also involved. With a malabsorption, however, there are as yet no symptoms. This term just states that a substance cannot be absorbed. What happens to the substance or how the body deals with it further cannot be deduced from this term.

"**Intolerance**", in the medical field, just means that something is incompatible. A substance is for example not being properly absorbed by the body – thus malabsorbed – and generates symptoms as a result. This means that the body is reacting to the substance that it cannot absorb properly, and does not tolerate it.
In short, this means: a malabsorption becomes an intolerance as soon as there are symptoms. And that is when you usually go to the doctor.

FROM THE PATIENT'S POINT OF VIEW:
The difference between these terms is thus in the detail and is normally irrelevant

for those affected. This means that the terms are used on websites or in books synonymously. Experience shows that most doctors are also unclear about the difference. This is also because this detailed differentiation is relatively new and often only available to experts.

The same applies to lactose intolerance: lactose maldigestion is the same as lactose intolerance. In this case, however, there are even more terms – which all mean the same: milk sugar intolerance, lactose malabsorption, lactase deficiency syndrome or alactasia. Different terms that in principle all mean the same.

FROM THE MEDICAL POINT OF VIEW:

For a precise diagnosis you must of course separate these terms. Doctors and scientists who are dealing intensively with this subject have to differentiate here. The differences are, however, irrelevant for the patient. A maldigestion can result in a malabsorption and this can then – though not necessarily – lead to an intolerance. This means: the substance is poorly digested, cannot be absorbed and then causes problems.

This means that there can be patients who do in fact have fructose malabsorption – thus the fructose is not being properly absorbed – but because they have no noticeable symptoms they do not have an intolerance. This, however, seldom occurs in medical practice because patients mainly attend when they have symptoms and thus already have an intolerance.

You often hear in medical circles that men in particular do not like to talk about their digestive problems. They thus have symptoms but won't admit it. The borderline between malabsorption and intolerance is thus extremely blurred in such cases. Quite apart from this, a malabsorption should also be treated because it could lead – even if the patient hardly notices – to further problems and worsen over time. Attention should certainly be paid to this in cases of multiple intolerances or also with patients with impaired self-perception!

In the diagnosis and in medical correspondence the terms should be correctly itemised where possible; in communications with the patient, however, definitions should be used that are clear and not couched in medical terminology.

Irritable Bowel Syndrome

Many patients, especially women, are given a diagnosis of Irritable Bowel Syndrome (IBS). This clinical picture is ranked among the functional intestinal disorders. The symptoms are very similar to those of fructose or lactose intolerance, which is why intolerance patients are often diagnosed – wrongly in this case – with IBS. In the case of IBS, however, the symptoms are not dependent on the food that has been ingested and are mostly influenced additionally by psychological factors. In practice it is not possible for those affected to distinguish between the two, also because, especially in the case of dietary fructose intolerance, the symptoms can appear with a considerable time delay. If you have been given a diagnosis of IBS, thus, you should insist that you get a precise differential diagnosis from your doctor and in this way eliminate other intestinal illnesses. This is especially the case when the symptoms persist after the elimination diet.

3. SUGAR AND SUGAR SUBSTITUTES

In order to get through the elimination diet successfully it is necessary to take a closer look at the different sugars and sweeteners. Here below we will get to know a couple of other sugars and sweeteners which we often come across on packaging or in the grocery store. We will also take a closer look at fructose itself. The chapter that follows is relatively complex. We have tried to make the subject as clear and as simple as possible.

Sugar alcohols

Let's first take a look at sugar alcohol and its close relatives. These are sweeteners or humectants (which keep things moist) that the food industry likes to use. A muffin without humectants would be dry in a couple of hours. With humectants, thus substances that keep the water in the product, the muffin stays soft for days. Some other substances are sweet, which means they can be used by the food industry to reduce the sugar content, which enables such products to be successfully marketed in this modern era as diet products or sugar-free products. But you should avoid having the impression that these substances do not also occur naturally. Many fruits, for instance, contain sorbitol or xylitol. The most frequent sugar alcohols are maltitol, xylitol and sorbitol. The –ol always means that it is classified chemically as an alcohol. Sugar alcohols should be avoided during the elimination diet; following the elimination diet you can certainly reintroduce some of the sugar alcohols that most patients can tolerate (that is xylitol or erythritol).

E-numbers

E-numbers like E965 are codes for chemicals which are approved for use as food additives within the European Union and Switzerland.

Maltitol (E965, Maltitol-Syrup) is a carbohydrate that is hard to digest. It has a low calory count. **Mannitol** (Mannite, E421) occurs in high concentrations in figs, some seaweeds, salsify, mushrooms and shitaki mushrooms. **Sorbitol** (Sorbit, E420) is contained, for example, in the fruits of the mountain ash, in raisins or in plums. It should be generally avoided in cases of fructose intolerance! **Isomalt** (E953) is present, for instance, in sugar beet. The food industry likes to use it because it is not only a tasty substitute for sugar but also has plenty of volume. Isomalt is also not recommended for those with fructose intolerance. **Lactitol** (E 966) does not occur naturally. This substance is often used as a sweetener but has a strong laxative effect and should be avoided in cases of intolerances.

Xylitol (E967) is found in birch bark but also in fruits such as plums. Xylitol is favoured for use in chewing gums and confectionary because, on the one hand, it is a powerful sweetener and on the other hand generates a cooling effect on the tongue – rather like menthol – and also works to prevent caries. Xylitol is generally harmless in cases of fructose malabsorption but can cause flatulence. For this reason it should be tested individually for tolerance! It should be avoided during the elimination diet. Xylitol is often used in toothpaste. But because you don't normally eat toothpaste, but spit it out again, such toothpastes are not a problem.

Erythritol is also a sugar alcohol. It occurs in many sugar-free products and some natural foods, for instance fungi or fruit. Most of the erythritol is reabsorbed in the small intestine with around 10% passing through to the rest of the digestive tract and being either excreted undigested or metabolised by bacteria. This sugar substitute is seen as relatively well tolerated in small quantities in cases of fructose intolerance. However, it should be avoided during the elimination diet and tested when establishing permanent eating habits.

Sugar

And now to the types of sugar. When we talk about sugar we usually mean the ordinary we use at home. But the word "sugar" is in fact just a collective term for all sweet-tasting saccharides. **Normal sugar** (household sugar / saccharose / sucrose / table sugar) is derived from sugar beet or sugar cane (when it is called cane sugar). "Sugar" is a disaccharide and consists of 50% fructose and 50% glucose. For this reason it is mostly tolerated in small quantities following the elimination diet – as we will see later. **Glucose** (Dextrose, grape sugar) is a sugar that can also be very well tolerated during the elimination diet. If you can't do entirely without something sweet then it provides a marvellous opportunity to satisfy the hunger for sweet treats. However, you should not consume too large a quantity of glucose because it can also act as a laxative, but only after consuming about 100g (3.5oz) per hour.

In general, you should leave out sweet things during the elimination diet, but every now and again it is ok to have something sinfully sweet. **Maltose** is composed of 2 glucose molecules. This means that, after the elimination diet, Maltose does not usually pose a problem. **Maltodextrin** is composed of 4 to 5 glucose molecules and is also ranked unproblematic.

Oligosaccharide is the general term for a chain of sugar molecules. This is mostly a chain of less than 10 molecules. The type of sugar is, however, largely undefined. **Polysaccharides** are even longer chains of sugar molecules (mostly more than 10). If this chain consists of fructose molecules then it is called **Oligofructose**. An example of this is **inulin**. This oligofructose is composed of around 100 fructose molecules and is often found in lists of ingredients. All these oligo- and polysaccharides, which are mainly composed of fructose, are also known as **Fructans**. Because they cause flatulence these are not tolerable in large quantities, though they usually are in smaller quantities – especially, too, because they cannot be broken down by the body and are thus to be seen as dietary fibre. This is an important point, because many of those affected are scared off when they see oligofructose or inulin on the list of ingredients. This, however, is unfounded because our bodies cannot break down these long fructose chains. Just the same, it also applies here to preferably try it out after the elimination diet. Since bacteria can break down these chains, tolerance depends on the individual intestinal flora.

Invert sugar (artificial honey) is a mixture of glucose and fructose and is mostly poorly tolerated.

HIGH-FRUCTOSE CORN SYRUP (HFCS)

You probably know this already: It is not good for you! HFCS is also called glucose/fructose (in Canada), glucose–fructose syrup in the European Union and sometimes you will find it under the name high-fructose maize syrup in some other countries. HFCS consists of approximately 55% fructose and 42% glucose. It is used instead of sucrose in the U.S. food industry. Reasons for this include governmental production quotas of domestic sugar, and an import tariff on imported sugar (e.g. from Cuba). HFCS is cheaper than normal sugar and because it is in liquid form, HFCS is much easier to process and transport. Health concerns about HFCS are that it may contribute to obesity, diabetes, cardiovascular disease, and non-alcoholic fatty liver disease (we will hear about that later). Whichever way you look at it, HFCS is not good for you, especially if you suffer from fructose intolerance. Food and drinks with added HFCS should be avoided!

Other terms for HFCS:
- glucose/fructose (in Canada)
- glucose–fructose syrup (in the EU)
- glucose-syrup (in the EU); even though it is called that, it often consists not just of glucose but also of a smaller quantity (less than 50%) of fructose)
- high-fructose maize syrup (in some countries)

SWEETENERS

And then there are the sweeteners. These include saccharin, aspartame, cyclamate or acesulfame K, among others. These substances are theoretically well tolerated in cases of fructose intolerance. But many patients don't tolerate them well so most experts advise against consuming too much of them. It is best to do without them, especially during the elimination diet. After that it is a good idea to test them out individually.

STEVIA

Stevia is a herbal plant with a strong sweetening effect that has been used for centuries in some regions of the world as a sweetener. It is very common in the U.S. and can be found in grocery stores or special health shops. Stevia has been approved in the EU since December 2nd 2011, under the name Steviol glycoside (E960) which is approved as a food additive for certain products. Stevia is well tolerated in cases of fructose intolerance, but be careful: many products use substrates or other sugars or sugar alcohols. This is why it is important to study the list of ingredients. In principle, Stevia is also well tolerated during the elimination diet.

ASSIMILATION OF SUGARS

Many of the sugars contained in our food are reabsorbed in the intestine with the help of carrier proteins, the so-called Glucose transporters (GLUT). The GLUT5 transporter, for instance, is responsible for fructose, the GLUT2 transporter for glucose. If there are only a few of these transporters available then the sugar involved cannot be assimilated quickly enough by the body, thus it is malabsorbed. As a result it is carried further down the intestine in the food pulp, where it is metabolised by intestinal bacteria. This gives rise to the typical intolerance symptoms. The GLUT5 transporter also reacts to other substances. Some sugar alcohols, such as sorbitol, block it, whereas glucose stimulates its activity. The individual quantities of fructose that are tolerated are thus very different. This lies mostly at the level of a few grams a day, but is also dependent on the other ingredients in the product being eaten.

4. AN OVERVIEW OF INTOLERANCES

The prevalence of food intolerances continue to rise. The number of those affected is increasing rapidly, particularly in continental Europe (presumably because there is a more scientific interest in these disorders). According to current figures, around 30 million people in the German language area are suffering from such an intestinal disorder. In most cases, the transport mechanism or enzymes in the intestine are impaired which means that certain carbohydrates cannot be properly digested. The symptoms range from bloating/flatulence and diarrhoea to nausea, fatigue and cases of depression.

The most common intolerances are **dietary fructose intolerance** (around 30%), **lactose intolerance** (around 15%-20% in people of European descent, approx 60-100% in people of Asian or African descent) and **histamine intolerance** (around 3%). There appear to be a particularly high estimated number of unrecorded cases of the latter in particular, however. There are significantly more intolerances whose classification and frequency in the continental European population is illustrated by the following table. There is not much data available about the frequencies of food intolerances in the U.S., especially because some intolerances – like fructose intolerance – are not yet well known in this region. We did a little survey with 1000 U.S. citizens in 2013. The data indicated that only 0.7% know about fructose malabsorption. This data can only be seen as a trend, showing that there isn't much awareness of fructose malabsorption in the U.S.

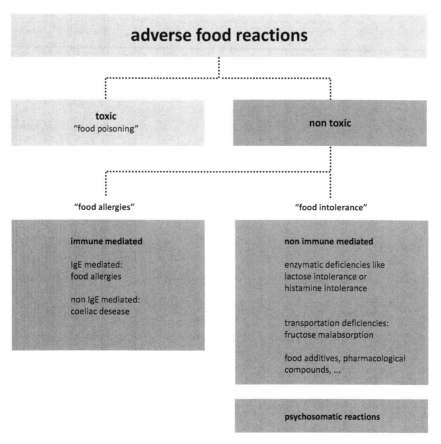

Fig: Adverse reactions to foods.

ANTIBODIES

Antibodies are also described as immunoglobulins, abbreviated as „Ig“. These immunoglobulins are „Y“-shaped and are composed of two long and two short protein chains. In chemistry, protein chains are classified according to the Greek alphabet. There are alpha chains, beta chains and gamma chains, for example.

Five different classes of such immunoglobulins occur in humans: IgA, IgD, IgE, IgM and IgG. These descriptions are according to the two longer protein chains. IgA, for instance, has two alpha chains, IgG two gamma chains.

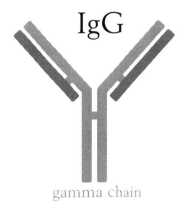

Fig: Immunoglobulin G with 2 gamma chains and two shorter protein chains at the upper ends of the Y. The antibodies connect to their respective targets at these ends.

These antibodies play a central role in the immune system. What is special about them is that anti-bodies have very specific targets. Thus, for example, when the viruses responsible for measles invade, we produce antibodies against this particular virus. These antibodies can be activated fast when there is a repeat contact with the virus and thus immediately prevent the illness. You are thus immune to this illness.

IgG is produced with a certain time-lag and then remains within the system for years (and sometimes for a lifetime). IgE is originally intended to combat parasitic diseases but also appears in the case of allergies, among others, and is formed very rapidly.

Food intolerances such as lactose or dietary fructose intolerance have absolutely nothing to do with these antibodies and cannot thus be diagnosed by means of IgG test procedures.
Only in the case of celiac disease, a very complex illness, do antibodies play an important role.

Antibodies can unfortunately turn against our own bodies. We still don't know why they do that. The result is the so-called "auto-immune diseases".

PROPER DIAGNOSIS OF DIETARY FRUCTOSE INTOLERANCE

The most common means of diagnosis is a **hydrogen breath test** (HBT).

The patient drinks a certain amount of a fructose solution (25g fructose dissolved in water) on an empty stomach. Afterwards the patient will be asked to blow several times, at certain intervals (normally every half hour), into a device that measures the hydrogen (H_2) levels from the air exhaled.

Since the fructose is not being properly digested there are bacteria in the intestines which produce hydrogen, short-chained fatty acids and CO_2. The hydrogen reaches the bloodstream via the large intestine and will consequently be exhaled through the lungs. By measuring the levels of hydrogen (which, by the way, does not itself cause any symptoms) it is possible to perform a diagnosis using this non-invasive breath test.

Apart from measuring the H_2 values, a record of the symptoms is an important part of the diagnosis. This is because not every person reacts the same way. Some patients don't produce any gas. Those persons are referred to as "Non-Responders". According to the most recent findings it is also necessary to measure the methane levels in these cases. Most physicians, however, do not have the proper medical equipment for this test and therefore it is important to pay close attention to the symptoms.

If symptoms such as bloating, abdominal pain, diarrhoea etc. appear during the HBT, then this is also a strong indication of intolerance.

The doctor concerned should also measure the blood sugar levels (except fructose testing) during the testing period. If an intolerance is present then the tested sugar is not absorbed into the bloodstream, resulting in the blood sugar level remaining the same. If there is no existing intolerance, then the blood sugar level will rise because the sugar is being absorbed into the system.

Preparing for the test

Your doctor should provide you with detailed information ahead of the test in order to be able to obtain a diagnostically conclusive result.

This includes:
- your needing to observe a short fasting period (12 hours before, no eating, just drink water)
- not smoking 12 hours before the test and during the test
- you should not have had a colonoscopy or an enteroscopy in the last four weeks before the test is administered
- you should not have taken any antibiotics in the last two (better four) weeks before the test is administered

Practical Tip:
On the day of your test, take the day off! If you are intolerant, then you will spend a substantial part of the day in the most private room of the house – the toilet – and suffer from severe symptoms, because you will have ingested a high dosage of the very substance you cannot tolerate on an empty stomach!

Where possible, your doctor should also determine other blood values via a blood analysis (folic acid, B12, serum analysis, lipase, zinc and iron)

5. LACTOSE INTOLERANCE

Lactose intolerance describes the inability of the organism to digest milk sugar (lactose) properly. Milk sugar is a so-called disaccharide and occurs in many dairy products. Normally it is broken down in the small intestine by an enzyme – the so-called lactase – into two single sugars (galactose and glucose) which can then be digested with the aid of GLUT transporters. This enzyme is either entirely or partially absent in people who suffer from lactose intolerance, thus the milk sugar cannot be broken down and further reabsorbed in the small intestine. Intestinal bacteria in the colon then process the milk sugar further.

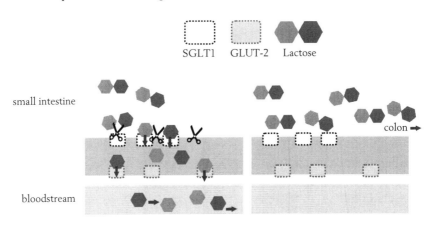

These intestinal bacteria form hydrogen (H_2), short-chain fatty acids and gases such as CO_2 or methane. By using the hydrogen (which in itself does not cause symptoms) it is possible to diagnose lactose intolerance by means of a pain-free breath test (H_2 breath test). The CO_2 causes flatulence while the short-chain fatty acids change the osmotic conditions in the intestine and lead to fluid entering the gut. The result is runny diarrhoea.

The individual amounts of lactose tolerated differ greatly. Most, however, are at around 1g (0.035 oz) a day. Over 20 per cent of patients with fructose intolerance also suffer from lactose intolerance. If you have not already been tested for lactose intolerance then you should definitely make an appointment for this through your doctor.

On the other hand, lactose intolerance goes hand in hand with fructose malabsorption in 80% of cases. The majority of celiac and gluten intolerance patients also suffer from lactose intolerance.

In the recipes at the end of the book we have tried for precisely this reason to avoid products that contain lactose. This means that all recipes are either lactose free or can be cooked without the use of lactose. An elimination diet is also important for lactose intolerance.

If the lactose intolerance is just a secondary symptom of fructose intolerance or the result of another reversible intestinal problem then there is a considerable chance of it healing itself. This takes some time and only works when you get a grip on the primary intolerance through dietary means. A systematic elimination phase is a great advantage here! However, if the lactose intolerance has a genetic cause, then it will not heal itself. A genetic lactose intolerance can be diagnosed by means of a simple blood test.

IS LACTOSE INTOLERANCE AN ILLNESS?

Mothers' milk is nutrition for very young mammals, thus infants. Adult animals do not drink milk and have no need to digest milk sugar – which only occur in mothers' milk. Since human beings are mammals, the same applies to them. Adult humans can no longer digest milk sugar. But it is the case that Europeans (and all those descended from them) can certainly digest lactose. Why?

According to some research, the North European human being developed the capacity to be able to digest lactose in adulthood about 7,000 years ago. The reason for this might lie in the fact there is a lack of sunshine (particularly in fall and winter) in the north of Europe. Vitamin D can only be formed with the aid of sunshine and is important for the formation of bones (calcium absorption). Consumption of milk is a good alternative for this but is unnecessary for people who live in sunnier climates.

This leads to the conclusion that lactose intolerance is not an illness, but rather more the norm. People who can digest lactose in adulthood are a genetic mutation.

But since these people are in the majority, our modern society concentrates on them. Because lactose is cheap and has a powerful lobby group, it is used in many products. The 15% of European descent and approximately 80% of Asian or African descent who suffer from lactose intolerance have to find their way in a western world full of lactose.

There are meanwhile many products that are labelled lactose free / dairy free, and there are whole ranges of products for the lactose intolerant. It is also important to note that many milk products are lactose free because of the way they are manufactured. In these, bacteria have already broken down the milk sugars during the maturing process. Cheese, in particular, can be made lactose free quite naturally in this way. Munster cheese, mature Swiss, cheddar or Gouda are very often naturally lactose free.

LACTOSE IN OUR FOOD

Products with less than 0.1g per 100g of food are defined as lactose free and thus well tolerated. Many with lactose intolerance can, however, tolerate a level of up to 1g per 100g quite well.

Cheese

When the carbohydrate content of the cheese is indicated, this is also an indication of its lactose level. Thus when it says Carbohydrates 0.0g (0%), then the cheese is lactose free. Starch is often added to grated cheese; in this case the cheese might be lactose free but the carbohydrate content is not zero! You can, however, mostly work this out from the information on the packaging.

The following table gives a broad overview. The values are meant as an indication since they can vary considerably because of the different processing and manufacturing methods.

Lactose level below 1g/100g	g/100g
Dark chocolate (75% Cocoa)	0-0.5
Brie cheese	0.5
Butter	0.5-1
Camembert cheese	0.5-1
Feta-Cheese (45 % fat)	0.5
Hard, mature cheeses (Gouda, Tilsit, Gruyeres, ...)	0-0.3
Parmesan, Grana Padano	0-0.1
Ricotta	0.3-1

Lactose level 1-5g/100g	g/100g
Buttermilk	4-5
Cottage cheese	4
Low-fat curd cheese	3-4
Mascarpone	2.5
Sour cream (15% far)	3.2
Curd cheese (20% fat)	2.7-4
Yogurt	1.2-4.5
Full-fat milk (3,6% fat)	4.6-4.8

Lactose levels above 5g/100g	g/100g
Ice cream	6-7 and more
Condensed milk	9-13
Skimmed milk powder	50
Skimmed milk	5
Milk chocolate	9-10 and more
Whey powder	73
Processed cheese, 45% fat in dry matter	6 and more

LACTOSE IS HIDING BEHIND THIS DESCRIPTIONS

Additives that contain lactose are often indicated obscurely on packaged foods. On the other hand there are ingredients that can be well tolerated although you might think they would not be. The following list contains some examples.

Containing lactose:
- Butter
- Buttermilk powder
- E966, Lactitol, Lactite
- Skimmed milk
- Cocoa paste
- Kefir (traditional kefir can also be low in lactose!)
- Kefir powder
- Condensed milk
- Lactose monohydrate
- Lactose
- Milk sugar
- Reduced fat milk
- Reduced fat milk powder
- Milk
- Milk products
- Milk powder
- Milk preparations
- Whey
- Whey products
- Whey powder
- Cream
- Sour whey
- Sour whey powder
- Chocolate preparations
- Sweet whey
- Sweet whey powder
- Full-fat milk
- Full-fat milk powder

Lactose free:

- Pure butter fat
- Clarified butter – made a fat from butter by removing water, milk protein and milk sugar; still tastes like butter
- Pure vegetable margarine
- Parve chocolate chips

MAY CONTAIN MILK INGREDIENTS

You often find this term used on packaging. This notification means that there are only very small quantities of dairy products to be found in the food. These quantities are sufficient to give rise to symptoms in allergy sufferers. However, these products are usually harmless for people with lactose intolerance because the amount of lactose they contain is far below the individual tolerance level.

LACTASE TABLETS: TAKING THE ENZYME YOU LACK

If you have an additional lactose intolerance, you should also leave out lactose during the elimination diet. Following the elimination diet it will be possible to eat foods containing lactose. The enzyme lactase, which breaks down the milk sugar, can be purchased in the form of capsules, tablets, soluble or powder form and be taken together with the meal. These compounds enable you to visit a restaurant or accept an invitation to eat out without problems. These little helpers are also unmissable on vacation.

Indication of the lactase content can be found in the FCC – the Food Chemical Codex – an unknown factor for the average consumer. This measures the purity of food chemical substances. The FCC was developed at the end of the 1950s in the USA.

General rule for lactase:
1g (0.035 oz) lactose is broken down by about 1000 FCC lactase (in vivo).

Lactase is harmless, which means that even an overdose can do no harm. It is thus better to take too much than too little! There are meanwhile a multitude of manufacturers but the pharmacy usually stocks only one or two sorts. For this reason you should always ask if there are other brands available or check out different pharmacies. It is generally advisable to test several brands and then to decide which one suits you best. There are tablets, sticks, powders or liquid lactase.

Important: The enzyme is deactivated above around 50 - 60°C (120-140°F), which means you should not open the capsules and stir the contents into hot dishes, or leave them behind in a car parked in the sun.

Be careful: Some lactase products contain sugar alcohols or other substances that are not well tolerated if you suffer from fructose intolerance. Most European manufacturers already changed their ingredients to tolerable ones, but in the U.S. these ingredients are still found quite frequently.

KOSHER AND LACTOSE INTOLERANCE

Kosher food provides an interesting opportunity for lactose-free food. "Kosher" means that the food has been prepared in accordance with Jewish food regulations. These regulations are extremely complex. What is important for those with lactose intolerance is that "dairy" food may not be eaten together with or for some hours before or after "fleischig" food that contains meat. It goes so far that not even the tiniest trace of dairy products may be eaten together with meat. In the orthodox Jewish tradition it goes even further, with separate refrigerators and pans for dairy products.

Besides the "dairy" and the "fleischig" foods, there are of course also "neutral" foods. These can be eaten with both of the other varieties and are thus free of any dairy element. These neutral foods are described as "parve" or sometimes "pareve".

Because orthodox Jewish communities observe these dietary rules extremely strictly, food has to be certified. The certifying authority issues a seal of approval that is printed on the packaging.

The "Orthodox Union" is one of the largest umbrella organisations of Orthodox Jewish communities and organisations in the USA. Their symbol (a U within an O) has additional symbols to match the certification.

- OU-parve: Neither meat nor milk. Tolerated in lactose intolerance
- OU-D: dairy, thus mostly not tolerated in lactose intolerance (D comes from Dairy). It can also mean that there are traces of dairy. For safety's sake the symbol should be taken to indicate: not tolerated.
- OU-M, OU-Glatt: strictly non dairy; which means can be tolerated for lactose intolerance.
- OU-F: "fischig", thus containing fish. This is mostly not tolerated by those with lactose intolerance but here, too, it may also mean there are only traces of dairy contained.

However, there are a vast number of kosher certifications. You often see a K inside a circle instead of a U. This is also an American organisation, "Organized Kashrut Laboratories". Here, too, it applies that as soon as a D or the word "dairy" appears besides the K, it contains (traces of) dairy products.

In the USA most grocery stores have kosher foods in a separate aisle. In many European cities there are also kosher supermarkets or restaurants.

Kosher and lactose intolerance

- Foods containing meat (but not fish!) must be lactose free
- Foods marked with "M", "glatt", "pareve" or "parve" must be lactose free
- If you get a meat dish in a Jewish restaurant or on a plane, then the sweet desert must also be lactose free. Cakes and other sweet dishes are mostly prepared with soy milk.
- Foods that are marked with a "D" or "dairy" are not necessarily lactose free – but could be; study the ingredients list!

6. HISTAMINE INTOLERANCE

Histamine is not a sugar but a biogenic amine. Put simply, biogenic amines are organic molecules that are responsible for a whole row of important functions within our bodies. Histamine also plays a central role in allergic reactions and inflammatory mechanisms. Histamine also works as an important regulatory factor in the digestive tract as well as in regulating the sleep-wake rhythm.

Histamine is generated within the body but can also be consumed in the form of food. It is only the latter that can give rise to histamine intolerance (HIT). Other biogenic amines can also cause problems with histamine intolerance, for which reason other foods containing large quantities of other biogenic amines count among those that are not tolerated. A "fish poisoning" or a "hangover" is in fact nothing more than a "temporary histamine intolerance". In these cases so much histamine (and other amines) has been ingested that even a healthy person can no longer deal with it. The consequences are the typical symptoms: headache, stomach ache, runny nose, nausea and hot flushes.

Histamine that is ingested as food is broken down in the small intestine by the enzyme diamine oxidase (DAO). The body wants to prevent too much of this substance being absorbed. Biogenic amines are also created when bacteria are living in food and are breaking it down – thus when a food either ripens or goes bad. For this reason it makes sense to have such an enzyme in the digestive tract. It prevents us suffering from a "fish poisoning" on a daily basis and makes it possible for us to keep food for a few days. In the case of histamine intolerance, the activity of the DAO enzyme is limited. Histamine that has been ingested is then not sufficiently broken down in the small intestine but is absorbed by the body and leads to undesirable effects there.

In a survey carried out by the "Society for Public Health" involving 141 subjects, the variety of symptoms were found to be distributed as follows: headache (38%), flushes in head and neck (36%;), stomach ache (31%), diarrhoea (26%), runny or stuffy nose (19%), flatulence and nausea (17%) and palpitations (12%). Less frequent, but still in more than 5% of cases, there were rashes, itchy skin, fatigue, dizziness and circulatory problems.

35

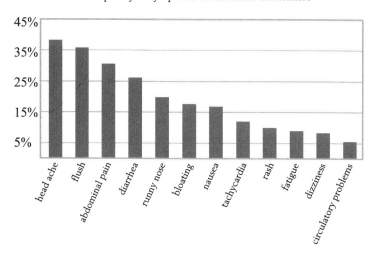

Fig: Frequency of symptoms in histamine intolerance in percentages

HISTAMINE INTOLERANCE – WHAT CAN YOU EAT, AND WHAT NOT?

There are foods which, as such, contain a negligible amount of histamine but which can release the body's own histamine. The following foods are seen as "histamine liberators" and thus cannot be accounted as tolerable, especially during the elimination diet: they include strawberries, some citrus fruits, tomatoes, kiwi and pineapple.

Alcoholic drinks, with red wine in particular, are seen as containing histamine or as DAO blockers, and thus also count as poorly tolerated. Foods with low histamine values but a high content of other biogenic amines are also seen as poorly tolerated. These include chocolate, cocoa, cured sausage, cured ham and bacon, and smoked sausage.

Fruit and vegetables are generally well tolerated; only processed products such as sauerkraut or pickles are seen as poorly tolerated. Despite this, there are also some kinds of fruit and vegetables that are seen as poorly tolerated because they contain high values of other biogenic amines. These amines are also poorly tolerated. These include spinach, bananas, pineapple, papaya, raspberries, pears, pulses, wheat germ and some nuts.

Alongside the usual problems such as, for instance, individual tolerance, the storage of food plays a major role in histamine intolerance. Freshly caught fish, for instance, is low in histamine, but if the same fish is stored without refrigeration its histamine content rises within a couple of hours, and a few hours after that it is full of histamine. In cases of histamine intolerance, fresh produce is always preferred.

NICE AND COMPLICATED!

I can understand if you are now thinking that the whole thing is far too complicated to ever be able to eat and live normally again. You really have to be an expert in nutrition to see the wood for trees!

But the good news is: it's not as bad as it looks!

In a major research project, we have had 109 different foods rated according to their individual tolerability. The resulting tolerability index has the advantage that the foods have been evaluated at a typical storage time and with the average state of processing. We then compared the results of this survey with intake recommendations and other scientific data, and were thus able to draw up a table that evaluates many foods according to their tolerability. In doing this, we found that some of the old food recommendations were incorrect. Raspberries, green beans and papayas were seen as poorly tolerated in cases of histamine intolerance. We were unable to confirm this in our research; on the contrary, papayas were mostly classified as well tolerated – after the elimination diet. Citric fruits also appear to be better tolerated than was accepted up to now. Despite all the tables, the most important maxim, and not just with histamine intolerance, is: always pay attention to your individual tolerance levels!

TABLE WITH TOLERATED AND POORLY TOLERATED FOODS

The table is ranked according to the degree of tolerance. There is another version of this table ranked in alphabetical order at the end of the book on page 134.

☺ well tolerated | ☺ sometimes tolerated – individual testing during the test phase recommended | ☹ poorly tolerated | ED = elimination diet | PD = permanent diet

Food	ED	PD	Food	ED	PD
Potato	☺	☺	Celeriac	😐	😐
Lettuce	☺	☺	Grapes	😐	😐
Rice	☺	☺	Onions	😐	😐
Courgettes	☺	☺	Pork	😐	😐
Chicken (without skin)	☺	☺	Coffee	😐	😐
Endive	☺	☺	Fruit teas, fresh	😐	😐
Lamb's lettuce	☺	☺	Mushrooms	☹	😐
Blueberries	☺	☺	Savoy cabbage	☹	😐
Pumpkin (Hokkaido)	☺	☺	Garlic	☹	😐
Dandelion leaves	☺	☺	Bell peppers (green)	☹	😐
Carrots	☺	☺	Chanterelle mushrooms	☹	😐
Sweet potatoes	☺	☺	Plums	☹	😐
Watermelon	☺	☺	Porcini (Ceps)	☹	😐
Broccoli	☺	☺	Corn (tinned)	☹	😐
Chicory	☺	☺	Bamboo shoots	☹	😐
Chinese cabbage	☺	☺	Red cabbage	☹	😐
Fennel	☺	☺	Green beans	☹	😐
Cucumber	☺	☺	Peas	☹	😐
Fresh corn, cooked	☺	☺	Hoseraddish	☹	😐
Asparagus	☺	☺	Raisins	☹	😐
Sugar melon	☺	☺	Pears	☹	😐
Beef	☺	☺	Chickpeas	☹	😐
Apple	😐	☺	Tuna, fresh	☹	😐
Cauliflower	😐	☺	Sodas, diet	☹	😐
Redcurrents	😐	☺	Aubergine	☹	😐

Food	ED	PD	Food	ED	PD
Prickly pear	☺	☺	Avocado	☹	☺
Peach	☺	☺	Banana	☹	☺
Leek	☺	☺	Dates, dried	☹	☺
Radish	☺	☺	Lima beans	☹	☺
Beetroot	☺	☺	Mandarin / Tangerine	☹	☺
Gooseberry	☺	☺	Soy beans	☹	☺
Egg	☺	☺	White cabbage	☹	☺
Apricot	☺	☺	Malt beer	☹	☺
Artichoke	☺	☺	Figs, dried	☹	☺
Blackberry	☺	☺	Limes	☹	☺
Sweet chestnuts	☺	☺	Spinach	☹	☺
Pomegranate	☺	☺	Lemons	☹	☺
Kaki	☺	☺	Cocoa powder	☹	☺
Cherry	☺	☺	Spirits, distilled	☹	☺
Kohlrabi	☺	☺	Pineapple	☹	☹
Lychee	☺	☺	Strawberries	☹	☹
Mango	☺	☺	Pickled cucumber	☹	☹
Okra	☺	☺	Grapefruit	☹	☹
Black salsify	☺	☺	Kiwi	☹	☹
Salt water fish (not tuna!)	☺	☺	Orange	☹	☹
Fresh water fish	☺	☺	Tomato	☹	☹
Honey	☺	☺	Beer	☹	☹
Figs	☺	☺	Energy drink, sugar-free	☹	☹
Raspberries	☺	☺	White wine	☹	☹
Coconut milk	☺	☺	Tuna, tinned	☹	☹

Food	ED	PD	Food	ED	PD
Mangold	☺	☺	Energy drink with sugar	☹	☹
Papaya	☺	☺	Sauerkraut	☹	☹
Parsnip	☺	☺	Wheat beer	☹	☹
Rhubarb	☺	☺	Red wine	☹	☹
Brussels sprouts	☺	☺			

TREATMENT WITH TABLETS IN CASES OF HISTAMINE INTOLERANCE

In principle, there are two ways of dealing with the excess histamine.

There is now the option, in cases of histamine intolerance too, to make up for the lack of the DAO enzyme by taking it in tablet form. You take one or two tablets before the meal. This has to be tested on an individual basis. It is also recommended that the tablets only be taken when absolutely necessary, for instance when on holiday or when eating out in a restaurant. Important: the enzyme preparation should be kept at room temperature and must be taken as a whole capsule because otherwise the DAO would be deactivated in the stomach.

 Scan this QR code to see where you can buy these products.

Alternatively you can take anti-histamines. These are medications that block the histamine receptors and are also used in cases of allergies. By blocking the histamine receptors, the effect of the histamine is reduced but the histamine itself is not broken down! These anti-histamines are medication and should be prescribed by a doctor (EU), they are available without prescription - over the counter - at UK pharmacies and American drugstores.

7. FRUCTOSE MALABSORPTION

FRUCTOSE – WHAT'S THAT?

Fructose is a monosaccharide (simple sugar) that can be found in our food in three different forms. As free fructose, as a part of our table sugar (sucrose), and as a part of the so-called oligo- and polysaccharines, the fructans. One of these, for instance, is the oligofructose that often appears on the list of ingredients. These fructans are not broken down by the body; as roughage, they get down to the bacteria which then metabolise them in the colon. This results in short-chain fatty acids, hydrogen and CO_2. Consuming too much of these fructans can thus cause intolerance symptoms in anyone, such as flatulence, diarrhoea and nausea. Recently the description "oligosaccharide intolerance" has become fashionable in Germany. But this description is misleading, because this is not about an intolerance in the usual sense of the word. The enzyme tablets on offer can help you digest such foods with fewer symptoms, but this is not about a classic intolerance.

Free fructose means that the fructose (fruit sugar) molecule exists alone and is thus not chemically bound to other sugars. Fructose or fruit sugar occurs, as the name suggests, in fruits, thus in fruit and vegetables. And it can occur in bound form, for instance as a part of table sugar (sucrose). This consists of one molecule of fructose and one molecule of glucose. These two sugars are bound together and have to be broken up in the intestine, because they can only be absorbed individually. This is done by an enzyme called sucrose-isomaltase. This means that a molecule of household sugar is converted in the digestive system into one molecule of free fructose and one molecule of free glucose. Sucroser, by the way, is not only to be found in the kitchen cupboard but also occurs naturally in fruit and vegetables. A pineapple, for instance, contains around 8g of sugar and a banana can even reach a level of 10g of sugar per 100g of fruit. One of the usual soft drinks has about the same sugar level.

What happens now to those two free simple sugars in the intestine? The fructose is usually absorbed by the body while in the small intestine, via the GLUT5 transporters, the glucose via the GLUT2 or the SGLT-1 transporters.

How does fructose malabsorption work?

In the case of so-called fructose malabsorption, the **GLUT5 transporters** are only partially functioning. The free fructose cannot thus be assimilated and then passes together with the food pulp into the colon where the bacteria that live there process it. Here too, the result is fatty acids, hydrogen (H_2) and CO_2. The hydrogen, which, by the way, does not cause any symptoms, passes through the intestinal wall into the bloodstream and is eventually exuded through the lungs. This means that the hydrogen can be used for diagnostic purposes through the use of an H_2 breath test (see "Proper diagnosis of dietary fructose intolerance" on page 24). The rest of the metabolic products of the bacteria cause the typical dietary fructose intolerance symptoms. These include flatulence, abdominal cramps, diarrhoea, acid reflux and nausea. But they can also lead to constipation, zinc and folic acid deficiency, or even the NASH syndrome. The latter is fatty liver disease. NASH stands for None-Alcoholic Steatohepatitis, thus a fatty liver inflammation that is not caused by over-use of alcohol.

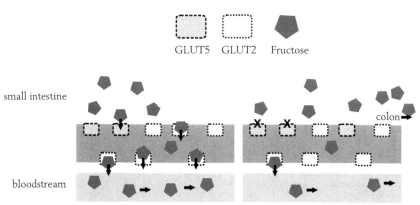

Fig: The way fructose malabsorption works.

Besides these physical symptoms, it is important not to forget the psychological aspects. Most of those affected, who have often been fighting the symptoms for years, retreat and limit their social contacts. They don't like to leave home (unless they know the precise location of the next clean toilet) and are often described by their social contacts as "long-term sick". Untreated fructose intolerance can even lead to depression.

The positive side is: as soon as you know what it is you are suffering from, the sooner you can do something about it. And make a start with the elimination diet.

You will see that you feel much better once you have successfully mastered the elimination diet and have got a proper grip on your dietary plan.

But before we take a closer look at this elimination diet, we would like to take a closer look at some of the basics with regard to fructose malabsorption. After all, to quote the classics – **know thy enemy**.

BASICS OF DIETARY FRUCTOSE INTOLERANCE

We have already established the difference between malabsorption and intolerance. But in some special cases of fructose intolerance there is one more difference. There is also **hereditary fructose intolerance (HFI)**, which is a very unusual hereditary form of the disease. A lack of the enzyme Fructose-1-phosphate-aldolase gives rise to damage to the liver and kidneys and to hypoglycaemia. In this case, the fructose is absorbed without a problem via the GLUT5 transport system, but then cannot be properly broken down by the liver. The illness already becomes apparent at a very young age, from the time a child is fed a supplementary diet.

The terms "**fructose malabsorption**" and "**fructose intolerance**" are used very frequently in the public domain for "**dietary fructose intolerance**". This book does not deal with hereditary fructose intolerance! For a better understanding of all terms concerning food intolerances please read the chapter "The difference between Malabsorption and Intolerance" on page 12.

Glucose improves the absorption of fructose in the small intestine, which means that it raises the tolerance level of fructose in patients who have fructose intolerance. Since glucose is reabsorbed significantly faster than fructose, foods with a high glucose component are generally better tolerated than foods containing equal quantities of glucose and fructose. Sorbitol and sugar alcohols reduce the tolerance of fructose because they impede the GLUT5 transporters. Foods that contain large amounts of sugar alcohols are thus seen as poorly tolerated.

Problems – Tables for Fructose Intolerance

What are Fructans?

Fructans are long chains of fructose molecules that are mostly not broken down in the body and are thus seen as roughage. Bacteria in the intestine, however, can metabolise the chains and this can lead, for instance, to flatulence.

Many food lists based on this theory have been launched in the past few years in Europe, in which fruit and vegetables are listed in accordance with their fructose-glucose relationship and quantities per 100g. In these, attention is always paid to the total-fructose, total-glucose and the sugar alcohols. Fructans are taken into account in hardly any of the tables. Neither have there been tables up to now that take individual tolerance into account. With dietary fructose intolerance, individual tolerance is also very important. This is why we at the "Society for Public Health" launched a research project in 2011 in which 109 foods were assessed by those affected in terms of their individual tolerance. The result of this comprehensive research project is the tolerance index which we have included in the tables in this book.

Many foods which, according to the existing tables, were supposed to be poorly tolerated were found by some of those affected who took part in our research to be very well tolerated. The same applies the other way around. Thus some foods were not tolerated which, according to the existing tables, should have been well tolerated. One example of this is the tomato. Raw, it contains per 100g around 1g of glucose, 1.3g of fructose, 0.1g of normal sugar, 78mg of fructans and 13mg of sugar alcohols. It should thus also be reasonably well tolerated in cases of fructose intolerance. In our research project we were able to show, however, that many of those involved had a poor tolerance of tomatoes.

Another example of the problems with such tables is the natural variables. In papaya we found fructose values between 0.3 and 4g of fructose as well as between 1 and 3.6g of glucose. Despite this the papaya is shown on most tables as being well tolerated. We were able to show in our research project that papaya is borderline.

It is often not nearly as well tolerated as the lists claim.

To sum it up: **in fructose intolerance it is also a matter of individual tolerance.** Tables can help in finding the right food for the test phase, but you will have to try out the different foods for yourself! Our research project also helped identify foods for the elimination diet. They form the basis for the tables contained in this book.

8. ELIMINATION DIET

Following the diagnosis, it is important to observe a so-called elimination diet. Since the diagnosis often comes after years of suffering and many miss-diagnoses, the intestine has been accordingly damaged. The good news is that our intestine recovers remarkably quickly if you allow it 2 to 4 weeks rest. This "rest" is known as the elimination diet. But so soon after the diagnosis, hardly anyone has had the time to get involved with nutrition, to think about fructose or lactose or histamine levels. Most patients who are freshly diagnosed feel completely lost at that moment and are afraid there is nothing left that they can eat.

It really is difficult to carry through such an elimination diet correctly without help. And it is just this observance of an elimination diet that is the key to an improvement in symptoms and to regaining your quality of life. We have felt it up close and personal ourselves and can tell you from our own experience: 100% is not enough to describe how much better you can feel if you feed yourself the right food! Look forward to it!

EATING AND FASTING

In our time and in the developed world we are used to having food always available. There is no famine close to where we live, nor is there seasonally limited availability. In addition, food is becoming more and more industrialised, which means that other substances are being added in order to make food keep longer, shine more, weigh more (at the same price), be lighter in texture and just to look better. Inevitably, quality and naturalness decrease while quantity increases. Over the past 60 years the diseases of civilisation have increased rapidly. Obesity, diabetes or raised fat or cholesterol levels are just some examples. Some types of cancer, colon cancer in particular, are associated with the high meat content of our diet. Vegetarians are significantly less affected. Now you have been diagnosed with fructose intolerance, it will be almost impossible to follow vegetarian diet - at least, not at the start of your journey.

The concept of fasting exists in almost every culture. Fasting, however, does not mean going hungry, but is about a temporary limit on what you eat and mental concentration on nutrition. People who fast regularly say they have a significantly better quality of life, more energy and more pleasure. Even when the first few days of fasting are not always easy, it all pays off!

Clearing out the intestine, letting the digestive system settle down and thinking about your own nutrition are the basic ingredients for successful fasting.

THE SITUATION FOLLOWING THE DIAGNOSIS OF FRUCTOSE INTOLERANCE

The stories I have heard over the last few years from those who are affected are similar in many ways and also reflect my own story. The problems mostly sneak up on you; you can't really say when the intolerance began. You have often been through "doctor marathons'", real "doctor-hopping". Many people end up with healers or other alternative forms of treatment, even if they do not believe in them. Quite often it is claimed that those affected have psychological problems and they are given the tip: eat more fruit and vegetables. At the end of my diagnosis marathon I was still eating an apple a day (because it keeps the doctor away...) although my body was telling me: cut it out! I was depressive, hardly left home and had just about lost the will to live.

We have asked people who use the german food intolerance network website to describe their personal history for this book. Some of their stories follow. These personal experiences are meant to give you the message: **You are not alone!** Many others have felt the same as you are feeling now.

EVA'S STORY

In the spring of 2011, after 15 years of abdominal pain, nausea and chopping and changing doctors, I was diagnosed with fructose malabsorption. Together with the diagnosis, the doctor instructed me to eat completely sugar and fructose-free for 2 to 3 weeks. Even though I was happy to have found a reason for my symptoms, the immediate question was how to make that work. Sugar is in absolutely everything, I thought. After several days I realised that this was not the case. With the help of my mother, who loves cooking, and some tips from various forums, I found plenty of tasty recipes and was amazed at how soon I started to feel better. Now, just over a year after the diagnosis, I am better than ever. I know what I have to eat, what does me good and what I have to be careful with. My friends and relations have also adapted to my particular eating habits so that there is nothing to prevent us from cooking together.

By eating foods that you can't tolerate, you damage your own intestines. Because this has mostly been going on for years, the whole intestinal trace has suffered considerably. In most cases, however, this is reversible and it thus normalises. Our intestine can stand a lot, but we also put it to the test. And that, although it is one of our most important and especially one of our largest organs. The intestine is around 8 meters (9 yards) long and has a surface area of around 500 square meters (600 square yard). Compare that to the ground area of your home!

In summer, we protect our skin with sun cream and we wear sunglasses to protect our eyes and helmets to protect our heads - but we do not protect our intestines! On the contrary, we cram them full with all kinds of sugars, alcohol and fats. And, if we are to believe the commercials, we eat a probiotic yoghurt every day. These are mostly full of fructans and sugar or even fructose, and if you also have an additional lactose intolerance then – bingo!

At the start of the healing process it has to be clear, then: your intestine needs a break during which it can regenerate. Your psyche needs a rest too. Stress has a negative effect on the digestive system. This means that the period of fasting should also go hand in hand with a certain calm. It has proved to work well if you start your elimination diet on a Friday. Then you have the whole of the weekend to concentrate on your food. It would of course be best if you could take a week off, but this will hardly be possible for most people.

The first week after the diagnosis is thus known as the elimination diet. Over the past few years this has become the most familiar term. You could also, however, refer to this period as Fructose Fasting or Lactose Fasting. In principle, it is all about leaving out the substances that are making your intestine sick and giving the intestine a chance to recuperate. This usually happens within 2 to 4 weeks, depending on how bad the damage is. What is important is that all the substances that make you ill are eliminated from the menu. If you have an additional intolerance then you should leave out those substances too – at least during the elimination diet!

The elimination diet is followed by the test phase. This is when you are testing out the amounts you can tolerate. This is because it is important, particularly in the case of fructose intolerance, not to avoid fructose altogether. Many of those affected can tolerate up to 25g (0.9 oz) of fructose per day quite well. If you were to leave fructose off the menu completely then you would just make your intolerance worse and you would probably get some deficiency symptoms on top of it. So during the elimination diet, leave out fructose as far as possible and then slowly introduce it back into your diet afterwards! This test phase lasts for 6 months on average. It can, however, take longer. I myself needed a year before I had my nutrition under control. However, at that time there were hardly any books or websites there to help me.

MARIE'S STORY

When, around two years ago, I first got a positive result from the tests for lactose and fructose intolerance, I was initially devastated. I had only researched on the Internet and thought I had found far too little information. No fruit. How will that work? I kept saying: I'll certainly end up with scurvy! I even went to nutritional counselling, but what I heard there was only what I had already found out from the Internet. The tip was: take vitamin pills for the rest of your life. Well... that wasn't my plan.

And how is it now?! I basically stick to the diet, but there are also regular exceptions. Sometimes more, sometimes less. According to what my body will allow. Some kinds of fruit, such as apples, are out. With others, small portions are tolerated. My husband has to eat the rest. But, basically, I eat fruit and vegetables every day and do not take vitamin pills. Chocolate or eating out in a restaurant or a piece of cake at a friend's house are all ok once in a while.

The initial period is the most difficult. You have to go your own way and learn to know and understand your body. After that you can live a perfectly normal life – with small limitations – and those around you hardly notice.

DEFICIENCY SYMPTOMS

Because the combination of food that you have been eating has damaged the intestine, some deficiency symptoms can occur in cases of fructose intolerance. Folic acid and zinc deficiencies, for instance, are often registered in fructose intolerance cases. **Zinc** helps the immune defences and also plays an important role in hormone balance. Zinc deficiency can be indicated by skin complaints (acne), increased susceptibility to infection, hair loss or the slow healing of wounds. Zinc occurs in meat, eggs, cheese and Brussels sprouts and has to be consumed continually because our bodies cannot store zinc.

Vitamins from the B group are known as **Folic Acid**. These vitamins are important for the blood corpuscles, cell construction, a number of metabolic processes and the nervous system. Folic acid is very unstable. It is destroyed by light, cooking or contact with air. When vegetables are cooked they lose up to 90% of their folic acid. If you wash chopped salad leaves, the folic acid is washed out. For that reason it is important to wash whole leaves of lettuce or other salad, and always to buy salad fresh. Salad that has been packaged, chopped and pre-washed contains practically no vitamins! The symptoms of folic acid deficiency include depressive moods, lack of concentration or irritability. As well as folic acid deficiency, patients with fructose intolerance sometimes have a low tryptophan levels. Serotonin, the **endorphin "happy hormone"**, is produced with the aid of tryptophan. If this is absent, then it can also give rise to depressive moods or even depression itself.

The body also reacts to such tryptophan deficiency with cravings for sweet things, because when you eat something sweet, insulin levels rise. This results in an opening of the blood-brain barrier which means that more tryptophan can be absorbed by the central nervous system. This results in an uplifting of the mood. But this triggers a vicious circle, because the sweet substance you have eaten probably contains fructose and was the actual cause of the trouble in the first place.

Attention: of course not every depression is caused by fructose intolerance. If you suffer from depression please go straight to your doctor!

Many of those affected are afraid that they will suffer from deficiency symptoms during the elimination diet. This is not the case! The elimination diet lasts for around 2 to 4 weeks; this period is too short to give rise to serious deficiencies. In the test phase, however, you should make sure you keep to a balanced diet because this phase will last for several months.

Elimination Diet	Test Phase	Permanent Diet
try to avoid all fructose and other sugars that are bad for you fructose fasting	find your levels of tolerance be creative and find foods that are good for you!	low fructose diet; do not avoid fructose! once a year: fructose fasting for 1-2 weeks
duration: 2-4 weeks	duration: approx. 6 months	

CHECK LIST FOR THE ELIMINATION DIET

- **Do I have other, additional intolerances?** 20% of those with fructose intolerance also have lactose intolerance!
- **Do I have an additional allergy?** Allergies are different from intolerances! You can be diagnosed by your doctor. For instance through a skin prick test.
- **Do I have deficiency symptoms?** A blood test by the doctor can establish whether there are any deficiencies. There are meanwhile preparations especially for those with fructose intolerance.
- **Are there other illnesses present that could make my fasting period dangerous?** This, for instance, refers to liver disease or eating disorders. Always start your elimination diet in consultation with your doctor!
- **Am I taking antibiotics or have I taken antibiotics within the last few weeks?** This is important because a disturbance of the intestinal flora can lead to additional digestive problems. If you have answered "yes" to this question, then ask your doctor about intestinal flora reconstitution products. Point out your intolerances, so that the products do not contain fructose, lactose, sorbitol or similar.
- **Do I have time to pay attention to my nutrition in the coming weeks?** It

makes no sense to start off the elimination diet during the Christmas rush or during other times of stress. This is because every time you break off the elimination diet, you have to start over back at the beginning!

- **Have I got enough cooking utensils?** You are going to cook for yourself. A basic set of equipment such as pots, pans and wooden spoons is necessary. If you are not a great cook, then please read the chapter entitled "The Little Cookery School"

TIPS AND TRICKS FOR A SUCCESSFUL ELIMINATION DIET

Coffee and sugar

If you only drink your coffee or tea with sugar, then substitute a Stevia product (inspect ingredients list!) or glucose for this. Other sweeteners are not recommended because they are also poorly tolerated by many of those affected. You can test out sweeteners individually after the elimination diet and then generally introduce them onto the menu. It would be even better if you left out coffee altogether. Caffeine generates a kind of stress situation in the body. Because stress usually affects the stomach, it is a good idea to generally leave out caffeine (also in form of sodas!). And it would be good to leave out cigarettes too!

Sweetening with glucose

Glucose is well tolerated and can be used during the elimination diet without a problem. Glucose is rapidly absorbed in the blood and has a strong effect on blood sugar levels.

For this reason you should be careful with glucose too and not use too much of it. If you use glucose in baking, then be aware that things brown more rapidly. You should adapt the recipe by lowering the temperature and extending the baking time.

Cook it yourself!

Always cook yourself! You have to come to terms with your nutrition, and you will not succeed with that if other people are cooking for you. When several people are there for a meal then they do not also have to eat fructose-free. We have collected together recipes that you can easily adapt so that all of you can enjoy them.

Small portions

Don't put a strain on your stomach. Prefer to eat less per portion but more often across the day. Eat regularly and concentrate on the food. That means you shouldn't be reading the newspaper or watching television while you are eating. Don't leave too long a gap between meals.

Food diary

Keep a food diary! There is a pro-forma page that you can print on the food intoler-
 ance network website, as well as an example you can copy here in the book (see page 125). If your problems remain during the elimination diet, then your doctor can perhaps use the diary to gather some important facts in order to help you.

What others think

We live in a culture where everyone is a self-proclaimed expert – especially when it's about food. You will see how many people offer you advice, whether you want it or not, or criticise your diet as such. Ignore these people. As we have already said, you should deal intensively and critically with the subject of food. You have to be the expert with regard to your own diet. What's good for you does not have to be good for anyone else, and vice-versa! You will learn to listen to your body. Because only your own body knows what is good for it, and thus good for you.

Eating disorders

There are many eating disorders out there and it seems that some intolerance patients who think too much about their food have a higher chance of developing an eating disorder. Please be careful and seek help if you should gain or lose too much weight! The intolerance or the food should not control your life!

Don't be a vampire!

Maybe it sounds stupid, but get out in the sun! Let the sun shine on your skin for a couple of minutes a day – without getting a sunburn. Breathe the fresh air and walk around in the countryside or in some park area. Sitting on the couch watching TV won't help you. Move your body and get some air!

THE ELIMINATION DIET BEGINS!

Here we go! Now we can start to bring your intestine back to its pristine state. First, have a close look at all the food packages you can find in your kitchen. Read the list of ingredients carefully. You will find that there are ingredients hiding in many products that are bad for fructose intolerance. Throw these products away or give them to someone else. The best thing is to organise a shelf in the refrigerator and one in the kitchen cupboard exclusively for you and the products you use. This is especially an advantage when you have a family.

The following ingredients are bad for you during the elimination diet and should be avoided (this list does not claim to be complete; as mentioned above, the E-numbers are used in the European Union and Switzerland).

- High Fructose Corn Syrup, Corn Syrup (any kind of syrup)
- evaporated cane juice, cane juice
- Fructans
- Fructose
- Isomalt, E953
- Lactite, E966
- Maltitol, E965, Maltitol-Syrup
- Mannite, E421
- Erythritol
- Oligofructose
- Polysaccharide
- Sorbitol, E420
- Xylitol, E967
- Sugar, domestic sugar, table sugar, saccharine, sucrose, liquid sugar, cane sugar

Be careful when a packaging is marked "fructose free" or "sugar free"

Recently the food industry in Europe has become aware of people with fructose intolerance. Increasingly, you can read "without fructose" or "fructose free" on the packaging. You have to be very careful with this! The devil is in the detail: sugar, thus saccharine, is split in the intestine into glucose and fructose. 10g of sugar is thus composed of 5g fructose and 5g glucose. According to the law, "fructose" is something different from "sugar". This means that foods to which no additional fructose – thus free fructose – has been added may be labelled "fructose free", no matter how much sugar it contains. The law doesn't care what happens to the sugar inside the body – which is also legitimate. And so long as it is outside the body, sugar is just "saccharine" and not "fructose". In the US "sugar-free" products are very common. They are normally sweetened with sugar alcohols and thus bad for people with fructose intolerance. Thus with these kind of products you have to study the list of ingredients very carefully, paying special attention to the total amount of sugar and sugar substitutes, in order to avoid any unpleasant surprises.

If you also suffer from lactose intolerance then you also have to avoid the following ingredients:
- Butter
- Buttermilk powder
- Lactitol, E966
- Skimmed milk
- Cocoa paste
- Kefir
- Kefir powder
- Condensed milk
- Lactose Monohydrate
- Lactose
- Milk sugar
- Low-fat milk
- Low-fat milk powder
- Milk
- Dairy products
- Milk powder

- Milk preparations
- Whey
- Whey products
- Whey powder
- Cream
- Sour whey
- Sour whey powder
- Chocolate preparations
- Sweet whey
- Sweet whey powder
- Full-fat milk
- Full-fat milk powder

Lactose free:
- Clarified butter
- Concentrated butter
- Vegetable margarine
- Parve margarine

FOOD LIST WITH TOLERABLE FOODS DURING ELIMINATION PERIOD

The tables have been composed on the basis of our above-mentioned research project together with experience gathered over the past few years. Those products marked with a superscript L should be avoided if there is an additional lactose intolerance.

In these tables, we have deliberately omitted fructose and glucose levels. The values are negligible and all these foods are suitable for the elimination diet. It is sufficient for you to deal with such values later, during the test phase. On page 65 you'll find a table with some more foods and at the end of this book on page 128 you will find another table, with about 140 foods in alphabetical order. Further tables, also containing glucose and sorbitol values, can be downloaded free from the food intolerance network website (just scan the QR code).

Vegetable products	Animal products
Avocado	Bacon*
Buckwheat	Beef
Celeriac	Cheese* (not processed slices!)
Cereal flour	Chicken
Corn starch	Cottage cheese* L
Cucumber	Cream L
Dandelion leaves & rucola	Egg
Fresh herbs	Fish
Lamb's lettuce	Ham* (not processed ham)
Lettuce	Milk L (cow, sheep, goat...)
Noodles* (semolina)	Natural yoghurt* L
Oils and fats	Pork
Potatoes	Bacon*
Rice	
Sour dough bread*	
Spinach	
Vinegar* (herb and apple vinegar)	
White bread*	

Table: Foods that can be tolerated during the elimination diet. Products marked with a superscript L mostly contain lactose, products marked with a * may contain sugar or other additives. Please inspect ingredients list.

This table is the product of years of experience together with a research project with over 800 participants which we carried out in 2012. In this research project we discovered that certain foods are tolerated differently from the way they are portrayed in the current literature. Rhubarb, papaya, apricots, bananas, grapefruit and mandarin oranges (tangerines) are often described as being well tolerated during the elimination diet, but that is not the case. These foods are very often not tolerated, which is why we have left them off the list. You can test these foods for your own individual tolerance level during the test phase. Potatoes are listed in some books as not being tolerated during the elimination diet. Our results show that this is not the case. Potatoes seem very well suited for the elimination diet. As a precaution, however, you should not try them on the first day but leave them until the second week.

WHAT YOU SHOULD NOT EAT

Besides the food additives and sugars already mentioned, during the elimination diet you should leave out wholemeal products, freshly baked bread and any foods that encourage flatulence, such as cabbage (brassicas in general) or beans. Carbonated drinks also cause flatulence. It is best to drink tap water or herbal teas (inspect ingredients list! Especially in the U.S. we found some teas with added syrups). You should also try to totally avoid alcohol and coffee. Depending on tolerance, you can drink one to two cups of coffee a day, but not more. It is best to drink coffee on a full stomach. The worst time for coffee is in the early morning on an empty stomach. Be careful with sweets and chewing gums. They almost all contain sugar alcohols and should thus be avoided.

For years there has been a stubborn rumour that you should also avoid toothpaste with sorbitol. That is nonsense because you don't eat toothpaste, you spit it out. And as long as the sorbitol does not get into the intestine then it is no problem at all for fructose intolerance.

In our book, however, we want to pay less attention to what you shouldn't eat and concentrate rather what you can eat!

Medication alert

If you have to take regular medication, then please speak to your doctor. Your whole digestive system will change because of the change in diet. This would mean that some medication can be better absorbed than it was before. The reverse is also possible. Your doctor might then consider adapting the dose you take. This subject is, however, extremely complex because you have to take so many factors into consideration. That is why we are only making a brief mention of it here, because it is something about which you must consult your doctor.

THE FIRST DAYS

The first days are certainly the most difficult. You have been used to a certain diet for many years, and are now making radical changes to this. Everything is new, and you probably still have symptoms.

At the start of the elimination diet you should mainly boil, steam and braise. Frying and roasting should be left for later. Rice and noodles are preferable to potatoes. Leave out vegetables and fruit entirely. Try noodles with egg, rice with parmesan, egg noodles with ham or fish or maybe chicken with rice or noodles. The best drink to accompany it is plain tap water or an herbal tea that does not irritate the stomach. As you can see, this resembles the kind of bland diet that is recommended if you have gastric flue.

If you also have histamine intolerance then leave out the parmesan and the fish. During the first few days also leave out bread unless you are baking it yourself and thus know exactly what is in it. You can eat some crisp-breads during the first few days, but you have to be cautious. Read the list of ingredients carefully! There are many of these types of bread that contain lactose or sugar. Rusk is not recommended because it contains a lot of sugar. As topping you can choose cheese, butter, or a cottage cheese with additions (but take care with both lactose intolerance and histamine intolerance) and fresh ham. You should avoid sliced sausage and processed ham because they often have sugar and other additives. Hard-boiled eggs are also an option. Don't be afraid of raised cholesterol levels – this phase only lasts two to three days and you can afford yourself a couple of eggs. Anyhow, recent research shows that eggs do not have the enormous influence on cholesterol levels as was claimed in the past.

In most cases there is a clear improvement after 3 days. The abdominal pain, the nausea and the diarrhoea mostly disappear first and the abdominal cramps and flatulence are less in evidence. I can remember precisely where I was, and when, the moment I realised how well I suddenly felt. I was standing at the lights on a pedestrian crossing, and felt good. When it turned green and I started to cross I felt really happy. Maybe that sounds a bit dramatic, but it is meant to illustrate how much your attitude towards life can be changed by eating the right food. I have heard similar stories from many of those affected.

ASTRID'S STORY

I have dietary fructose intolerance, and since I know about it I am much more conscious of how I cook and prepare most of my meals myself. I test things out at the weekend in order to keep expanding my list of foods. This means that I don't lose a day's work if it doesn't work out. Because I don't have to do without sweet things altogether, I cook with glucose; for instance cakes, cookies or jam. My family really enjoys this. Of course, I also bake and cook "normal" stuff for them. When I am shopping I always pay special attention to the sugar content of foods and I already have a long list of products I can tolerate.

Because I am now eating more healthily and paying attention to my diet, this also has a positive effect on my mood and my health. I am totally happy for days at a time when I have tolerated something 'new'. So it is about the many, if small, advances that keep on encouraging me and making me happy. I have developed a passion for collecting tolerated foods, and thus also of that feeling of success.

THE FIRST TWO WEEKS

You should already be feeling better. If you still have symptoms, don't despair. With some people it can last longer before the intestine has settled down. But please be extra careful not to commit any "elimination sins". If you have a craving for something sweet, try a glucose tablet. But here, too, pay close attention to the list of ingredients!

You can now start trying out other foods. You can now test potatoes or courgettes. Try some of the recipes in the recipes chapter. First try incorporating spinach, lettuce and cucumber into your menu. These products are rich in folic acid and are well tolerated. Start slowly – that means trying out one new thing a day. Don't put a strain on your body with a banquet! In the days to come, feel your way slowly into your new nutrition pattern but always keep in the back of your mind that you are fasting and giving your intestine time to recuperate. It can happen that during this period your intestine goes on the rampage. There are often reports of constipation or a very hard stool. That is normal and should adjust itself in the days to come when more fibre is introduced.

After two weeks at the latest you should be feeling better. If there is no improvement after two weeks then please go to the doctor soon with your food diary and discuss how to proceed. There could be a bacterial overgrowth or another illness that has not been recognised up to now.

Small Intestinal Bacterial Overgrowth

Many patients with fructose intolerance suffer from "Small Intestinal Bacterial Overgrowth" (SIBO).

This means that bacteria from the colon have infested the small intestine and are causing problems there. These bacteria have been able to pass through a kind of intestinal valve, the so-called ileocaecal valve, because the intestine is so inflated, and thus invade the small intestine where normally few of them live. The doctor should be able to diagnose this with the help of a further breath test with lactulose or by a more precise evaluation of the original test. It is possible to treat this with antibiotics and a restitution of the intestinal flora.

THE LAST TWO WEEKS

You can get a bit bolder during the last two weeks of the elimination diet. You can cook with larger quantities of the foods you have tolerated well. Try a few onions and garlic (never raw!), and also test bananas and tangerines, mushrooms or broccoli now. But all in small quantities and one after another. If you tried out all of them at once then you would be unable to deduce which one is causing symptoms. So you need to limit yourself to introducing one new ingredient per meal! Many of those affected finish the elimination diet after 3 weeks and start the test phase in week 4. The transition is certainly smooth. My experience of the end of the elimination diet was that I suddenly had a craving for apricots – although I had never been all that fond of apricots. So I went out and bought just one apricot, and ate it, and tolerated it. At that moment it became clear to me that this was the end of the elimination diet and that I had learned to listen to my body.

FRUCTOSE FASTING: ONCE A YEAR

It has been shown that it does you good to hold a fructose fast once or twice a year – even when you have got a firm grip on your diet. Despite this, you will continue to cross the line now and again. That is quite normal. We thus recommend that all "fructose professionals" take a fructose break of around two weeks, once a year. In our western culture, lent is probably the best time for this, particularly because during this period people don't ask silly questions and question your motives if you are fasting. On the contrary, people who fast during these periods are usually given respect and understanding.

9. THE TEST PHASE

Try out everything you fancy. But be really aware of the quantities, your symptoms and, especially, listen to everything your body is telling you. The time after the elimination diet is not a free-for-all! The intolerance has probably not been cured but your intestine has calmed down. Experiment with your diet and find your personal tolerance level! During our research into the tolerance index for foods one thing became very clear to us: there is no single food that is well tolerated by everyone. Even rice is indicated by around 2 per cent as being difficult to tolerate.

As we have said repeatedly, listening to your own body is the most important thing.

The main purpose of the test phase is to detect what and how much of it you tolerate, and what and how much of it does you good. We estimate a period of 6 months for this phase. The truth, however, is that you can't say precisely how long. In principle, you are always going to have to test because your tolerance levels will change, according to your personal sensitivity. It is perfectly normal for you to be able to tolerate foods on holiday that you can't eat at home. It is perfectly normal that you might have been eating courgettes, for example, every day and then, suddenly, find you cannot tolerate courgettes on one particular day. Tolerance depends on so many different factors that, in principle, it can never be nailed down precisely. Some of the variables are the degree of maturity, the type, the way it is prepared, stress, the composition of intestinal flora, infection, or your mood on the day.

But after around 6 months you should have your eating habits and your diet under control to such an extent that a normal life is possible.

TABLE OF WELL TOLERATED AND POORLY TOLERATED FOODS

The following table includes the foods involved in our research project and should support you during the test phase. There is an extended table in alphabetical order at the end of the book on page 128.

☺ Well tolerated | ☺ Sometimes tolerated | ☹ Poorly tolerated
ED = elimination diet | TP = test phase | PD = permanent diet

food	ED	TP & PD
chicken	☺	☺
rice	☺	☺
fish, fresh (not canned fish!)	☺	☺
Lamb's lettuce (corn salad)	☺	☺
potato	☺	☺
beef	☺	☺
egg	☺	☺
dandelion leaves	☺	☺
green salad (lettuce)	☺	☺
pork	☺	☺
zucchini / courgette	☺	☺
avocado	☺	☺
chicory	☺	☺
fennel	☺	☺
cucumber	☺	☺
chard	☺	☺
spinach	☺	☺
fresh sprouts	☺	☺
cep	☺	☺
eggplant	☺	☺
bamboo shoots	☺	☺
broccoli	☺	☺
coffee	☺	☺
parsnip	☺	☺
chanterelle	☺	☺

food	ED	TP & PD
sweet potato	😐	😊
canned fish	😐	😊
pickels	😐	😊
artichoke	😐	😊
mushrooms	😐	😊
chinese cabbage	😐	😊
peas	😐	😊
pumpkin (hokkaido)	😐	😊
lime	😐	😊
carrot	😐	😊
okra	😐	😊
celeriac	😐	😊
asparagus	😐	😊
papaya	😐	😐
banana	😐	😐
chestnut (maroni)	😐	😐
cauliflower	😐	😐
cocoa powder	😐	😐
chick-pea	😐	😐
coconut milk	😐	😐
horseradish	😐	😐
radishes	😐	😐
rhubarb	😐	😐
beetroot	😐	😐
salsify	😐	😐

food	ED	TP & PD
lemon	🙂	🙂
green beans	🙂	🙂
blackberry	🙂	🙂
fresh corn, cooked	😐	😐
blueberry	🙂	🙂
currant	🙂	🙂
prickly pear	🙂	🙂
lychee	🙂	🙂
corn, canned	🙂	🙂
mandarin (tangerine)	🙂	🙂
schnaps	🙁	🙂
soybean	🙂	🙂
raspberry	🙂	🙂
kohlrabi (turnip)	🙂	😐
beer, lager	🙁	🙂
red cabbage	🙂	🙂
grapefruit	🙂	🙂
kale	🙂	🙂
garlic	🙂	😐
green pepper, bell pepper	🙂	😐
brussels sprouts	🙂	🙂
tomato	🙁	🙂
watermelon	🙂	🙂
musk melon	🙂	🙂
apricot	🙁	😐

food	ED	TP & PD
strawberry	☹	😐
pomegranate	☹	😐
kaki	☹	😐
lima bean	☹	😐
gooseberry	☹	😐
fig	☹	😐
kiwi	☹	😐
orange	☹	😐
peach	☹	😐
leek (allium)	☹	😐
red wine	☹	😐
cabbage	☹	😐
white wine	☹	😐
onion	☹	😐
pineapple	☹	☹
brown ale	☹	☹
mango	☹	☹
sauerkraut	☹	☹
wheat beer	☹	☹
cherry	☹	☹
plum	☹	☹
raisin	☹	☹
apple	☹	☹
grapes	☹	☹
pear	☹	☹

food	ED	TP & PD
dried date	☹	☹
energy drink, diet (sugar-free)	☹	☹
energy drink, with sugar, fructose or HFCS	☹	☹
dried fig	☹	☹

Table: Toleration of foods in cases of dietary fructose intolerance.

10.   TIPS & TRICKS FOR PERMANENT DIET IN FM

In conclusion, a couple of helpful tips and tricks for your long-term nutrition. As we have mentioned, an annual fast does no harm – on the contrary, it is highly recommended.

BAKE YOUR OWN BREAD!

Learn to bake bread! The bread you buy often contains additives you cannot tolerate. When you bake your own bread, you know exactly what it contains. Baking bread is not easy and needs a bit of practice and patience. Your first attempt will probably not be a success, but with a bit of practice you will soon learn to bake good bread yourself. A bread baking machine is a useful investment (and saves a lot of hassle and frustration) and, with the current price of bread in the shops, it will pay for itself within a few months.

THE GLUCOSE TRICK

For most patients, glucose makes it easier for the small intestine to absorb fructose – thus when there is a molecule of glucose present in the small intestine for every molecule of fructose, most people have no problems with fructose. This differs, however, individually and depends on the number of functional GLUT5 transporters present. It also depends on the amount of fructose that reaches the intestine. In addition, the total fructose consumption per day has to be taken into account because you can only make a certain quantity of fructose more tolerable per day with the "glucose trick".

What is important is to know that the glucose is reabsorbed very quickly while fructose stays in the intestine for a relatively long time. This means that if you eat 1g of fructose and 1g of glucose then, after a relatively short time, there will again be a fructose surplus because the glucose has been absorbed faster. This is why it is advisable to consume more glucose than fructose.

But take care: do not eat too much glucose because that can play havoc with your energy balance. The "glucose trick" is something reserved for holidays and meals out.

TABLETS THAT MIGHT HELP

There are also meanwhile tablets that can help in cases of fructose intolerance. These products have been developed in Austria but are available worldwide. See our website for online shops where to buy the product.

The tablets contain the enzyme "**Xylose Isomerase**". This enzyme converts the fructose into glucose in the small intestine – but also glucose into fructose. In principle, what is happening here is the "glucose trick without the glucose" because the fructose that has been consumed is converted by this enzyme into glucose which is then absorbed. It is in the nature of the enzyme to always want to restore the balance between fructose and glucose. This means that if equal quantities of the two sugars are present that it stops converting fructose. But because the glucose is rapidly reabsorbed there is again an imbalance in the intestine, so that almost all the fructose gets converted. But this also means that, theoretically, consuming more fructose would suppress the working of the enzyme. However, the glucose is absorbed so rapidly that there is still an imbalance. This means: if you take the enzyme then you do not need any extra glucose.

Important: The enzyme is deactivated above 60°C (140°F), which means that you should not stir the enzyme into hot food or leave it in the car when you are parking in a sunny spot. Always take it according to the instructions in the leaflet provided.

———————

MARKUS'S STORY

Three years ago I was diagnosed with fructose intolerance. I then did a lot of reading and kept a strict diet for 4 weeks. I only really ate rice, noodles and eggs. After that I left out fructose as much as possible. A few months later I was reacting more and more strongly to fructose and was failing to tolerate all the tested foods. My doctor then told me I had made a mistake. You should not leave out fructose altogether; that only makes the problems worse because the intestine just gets used to it and reduces the fructose absorption even further. I have meanwhile reintroduced fructose into my diet and since then I have been feeling much better.

I can meanwhile even drink beer again! I still can't tolerate tomatoes, but perhaps that will change in time....

Do you have to eliminate fructose altogether for the rest of your life?

No! It is only during the elimination diet that you should avoid fructose as much as possible. After that, you can experiment with small quantities until you find your personal "dose". Recent research shows that eliminating fructose altogether in the long term just makes the problems worse. So you should certainly consume fructose, but only in quantities that you can tolerate!

How can I sweeten things if I have fructose intolerance?

Instead of honey or sugar you can use rice-syrup, stevia or glucose. Read the ingredients lists of those products carefully! However, you should not use any other types of syrup! Ordinary sugar is mostly only tolerated in small quantities because it consists of equal quantities of glucose and fructose. People who do not have lactose intolerance can sweeten with lactose (milk sugar), but this can also act as a laxative!

When can I eat fruit, and how much?

Fruit is best following a main meal and preferably in the afternoon. This means that breakfast banana is less well tolerated than a banana in natural yoghurt as a desert for lunch.

Soy milk, rice milk and other milk substitutes

You can go for milk alternatives, especially if you have an additional lactose intolerance. With soy milk, almond milk or rice milk, keep an eye out for added sugar. There are also products without added sugar. These are very well tolerated and are extremely suitable for cooking and baking. We frequently use rice milk in particular in our recipes.

Travelling with intolerances

Before you travel, read up on the local eating habits, for instance on the Internet. Consult the various forums and ask people there if they have visited that particular country or area and perhaps have some tips for you. Let's take Thailand as an example. When I first went there I took a pack of lactase tablets with me. They were used up quickly because the tourist menu was full of lactose. I wanted to buy some fresh tablets but because Thai people do not eat dairy products there was, of course, no lactase on sale. The pharmacists just looked puzzled. Then I started to insist on local food and kept away from the tourist traps. That meant I had no problems and was getting much better food. Another example is the USA: here you can buy lactase tablets everywhere in every shape and form.

Enzyme products for fructose intolerance and histamine intolerance are currently mainly available in the German language regions. But you can order them world-wide online. See our website for links to the online shops. Anyway, this means you should take a sufficient supply with you. It is also a good idea to take glucose (dextrose tablets) with you, at least for an emergency.

You can also, in consultation with your doctor, expand your travelling pharmaceutical kit with medication that will reduce nausea and bloating.

Airline meals

If you have lactose intolerance, I always recommend you order the kosher menu. Most airlines do offer a "lactose free" menu, but that is mostly a vegan menu. People with fructose intolerance have an even bigger problem with that. The kosher menu is in all probability lactose free (see section on "Kosher and Lactose Intolerance"), and it mostly tastes better than the normal in-flight meal. It is also a better choice for those with fructose intolerance because in our experience there is little use of high-fructose corn syrup and sugar alcohols. If you do happen to get a dairy meal, then you can always resort to lactase tablets.

It is thus perfectly possible to travel with intolerances. All you have to do is be a little cautious and get the right information.

OTHER INTOLERANCES

There are many other food intolerances, such as gluten intolerance or gluten sensitivity. Gluten is the generic name for certain types of proteins found in common cereal grains. About 1% of the population suffers from gluten intolerance or a more severe form, celiac disease. There is also wheat allergy. So that chapter is very complex and would be too much for this book. But we have a lot of information on line on our website, so if you suffer from any other intolerance, feel free to go to the food intolerance website at www.food-intolerance-network.com. Some recipes at the end of this book are gluten-free too.

11. COOKING MADE EASY

Can't cook, won't cook? Then this is the chapter for you. If you are a good cook please ignore this chapter!

Now that you have been properly diagnosed with a food-related intolerance, you have simply got to learn to cook for yourself. No excuses. Of course you can let someone else do the cooking for you, but you risk losing the battle. You have to start tackling your own eating habits. You have to know precisely what is in your food. As long as you don't know what you're eating there is no way you can learn to deal with it. Your target is to learn to eat well and live symptom-free without having to depend on others.

This chapter is thus for culinary beginners. Over the past years we have repeatedly staged cookery courses and I was simply amazed by how many people know nothing at all about cooking. That is why we are going to use this chapter to spell out the basics – things that are already understood by those who cook because they love it or because they just have to cook for their family.

COOKING UTENSILS

You need some basic equipment. This includes:
- 1 or 2 chopping boards
- Sharp kitchen knives
- 2 or 3 wooden spoons
- Ladle
- Turner for non-stick pans
- Non-stick frying pans – leave those without a non-stick surface to the professionals!
- 1 or 2 small saucepans (with see-through lids if possible)
- 1 large saucepan
- Whisk
- Can opener
- Fork and spoon – for tasting
- Sieve

- Big glass salad bowl
- Plastic mixing bowl
- 2 or 3 smaller bowls
- Salad spinner
- Empty, clean glass jam-jar with lid – you will need this for salad dressings – see recipes.
- Tea towels – always wash hot (at least 140°F / 60°C)
- A timer

A hand-held blender, a roasting tin, a steamer insert and a pestle and mortar are also useful to have. A hand mixer would do no harm. An ice machine or a sushi set could give you a lot of pleasure. A microwave oven will save you a lot of hassle (let alone a lot of washing up).

A COUPLE OF COOKING TIPS:

- Only use the right implements with a coated, none-stick pan. Metal implements scratch the pan's none-stick surface and render it unusable.
- Kitchen knives can blunt faster if you put them in the dishwasher. Be careful how you stack non-stick pans so as not to scratch the Teflon surface. Never put oiled wood (such as salad bowls) in the dishwasher.
- Always spin washed salad in the salad-spinner, because the dressing only attaches itself to dry salad. The dressing runs off wet salad, leaving you with a water-dressing mixture at the bottom of the bowl. Don't over-wash salad or vegetables.
- Keep it clean! Cooking in a dirty, untidy kitchen is not good for your health or your mood.
- Don't cook when you are very hungry, or in haste. That mostly doesn't work. Take time for cooking, especially when you are not really familiar with it.
- Don't be afraid to ask others for advice. If you know someone who is a good cook, then let them give you tips, or cook together sometime.
- Watch some cookery shows on TV. They are not just entertaining, but you can learn a whole lot from the real professionals.
- Don't be discouraged if things don't go right first time. Learn to laugh about it.

COOKERY BASICS

Braising and Steaming

This is the best way for you to prepare food now. It is kind to the food and to our much-abused digestive systems. The food goes into a pan with a little liquid (water or stock). The lid goes on tight. The food cooks mainly in the steam on a low flame. Important vitamins and minerals are thus preserved. It is most important that the temperature is not too high, otherwise the water will evaporate and the food will burn. This method is ideal for the start of the elimination diet because it is the gentlest method.

There are steamer inserts that fit into pans. They look like fold-up satellite dishes. These "metal umbrellas" fit most pans. They have a small base, mainly three small feet, so that the food is not swimming in water but is just cooking in the steam. This means that important ingredients are not washed out.

There are also cooking bags designed for the microwave. All you have to do is put the vegetables in the bag, without any added water, seal and cook for 2 to 4 minutes on full power. In some grocery stores you may get some vegetables ready-packed in such microwave bags, ready for cooking in the microwave.

You may also use both alternatives for your recipes. This means that the food is first fried briefly, then water is added and it is cooked further.

Frying and roasting

Frying means you are using fat, or preferably oil. The best way to fry something is to heat up the pan briefly, add a little (1-2 tablespoons) oil, turn the heat down to medium, add the food, and fry briefly until cooked. This results in flavours that give the meal a special taste.

It is important not to let the oil get too hot because this could result in by-products that are bad for your health. If the oil is smoking then it is too hot and should not be used. You should let it cool off and then dispose of it. Never, ever pour water or any liquid on hot oil; that could lead to an explosion and a fire. Never put wet food into hot oil for the same reason!

You should use heat-stable oil or fat for frying. This includes olive oil, coconut oil, sunflower oil or lard. Special salad oils and flavoured oils such as rapeseed oil, pumpkin seed oil or sesame seed oil should never be heated.

If you are using so much fat that the food is swimming in it, you call it deep frying. This is not the best means of preparation for you now, especially not during the initial days of the elimination diet.

Roasting happens in the oven. You will need to follow a recipe. Make sure the oven is up to temperature (which usually takes about 10-15 minutes) before you put the food in and set the timer. If you use the fan setting then you can lower the temperature a notch, or by 50°F (10°C).

Chopping and slicing vegetables

Top restaurants have many techniques for chopping and slicing vegetables. This has several reasons. On the one hand, it is about presentation, on the other about taste and flavour. Plants are composed of fibres and liquids. Depending on how a plant is cut, the liquid and thus the taste either emerges or remains within the plant. That, however, is not relevant for us now. Be creative! Cut up your vegetables the way that seems right for you. When you eat them you will know whether you want to slice them differently next time round.

PREPARATION OF CERTAIN BASIC FOODS

Cooking basic pasta or noodles

Fill a big, deep pan ¾ full with water. Put it on the stove and turn the heat on full. Put the lid on. (This will make the water boil faster and save on your energy bill). As soon as the water is boiling take the lid off and add a teaspoon of salt to the water. Take care, it will bubble up briefly. Now add the noodles and stir briefly with a wooden spoon. Turn the heat down, otherwise it will probably boil over and mess up your stove. Let the water simmer gently for the rest of the cooking time. You will find the time the noodles need to cook on the packaging. Set your timer. When the cooking time has lapsed, put a sieve in the sink and carefully drain the noodles into it. Take care – the steam that comes off is very hot and can scald! It's best to use oven gloves. The noodles can now be served up or prepared further. You can also put them back in the pan and add a few drops of oil, then shake or stir. Put the lid back on and they will stay warm while you prepare the rest. But DO NOT put the pan back on the heat!

Boiling rice

There are many, many ways of cooking rice. Wars have been fought over less. You can follow the instructions on the pack, but this is my (almost) fail-safe method. First make sure you have the right kind of rice. Do not attempt to boil pudding or risotto (round-corn) rice. Use a long-corn variety or basamati. Three-quarters fill a small pan with water and bring to the boil, as for pasta above. Add a little salt (optional; 1 teaspoon). You would be surprised how little rice you need to make a portion. Half a cup of dried rice will make two portions - yes, it really does. Add the rice, stir once, turn the heat right down, let it cool down to simmering and put the lid on. Set the timer to 10 minutes. If the rice threatens to boil over take the pan off the heat for a moment. When the timer goes off, drain the rice into a sieve, then pop it back in the pan, put the lid on, put it somewhere OFF the heat and let it stand for a few minutes or while you prepare other food to go with it. This method also works well for boil-in-a-bag. Again, use plenty of water, and let it rest a bit after you have drained it.

Boiling eggs

When you boil eggs, you can make them either hard or soft. The difference is simply in the cooking time. Put the number of eggs you need into the pan. Fill the pan with tap water until the eggs are well covered. Then put the pan on the stove and bring to the boil. (If you put the eggs into boiling water they are more likely to crack.) When the water starts boiling, turn the heat down to medium. Set the timer. The cooking time starts as soon as the water begins to boil. In general, a soft-boiled egg needs four to five minutes and a hard-boiled egg needs just over seven minutes. These times depend on the size of the egg and even on the altitude at which you are cooking. You will find your ideal time – and egg – by experimenting.

Cooking potatoes

There are many ways of cooking potatoes. This method is the one most suitable for use during the elimination diet.

Fill a big enough pan half full with water. You will need enough water to cover the potatoes. Put it on the stove and bring to the boil at full heat, with the lid on. As mentioned above, this means the water boils faster, saving your energy bill. Peel the potatoes as thinly as you can. Cut them into cubes of around an inch (2cm). As soon as the water is boiling, take the lid off and add a teaspoon of salt (optional). Take care, it bubbles more for a bit. Now add the potatoes, bring back to the boil and turn the heat down to medium with the lid back on. After about five minutes, test the potatoes with a fork. If they are still hard, they are not yet cooked. If the fork goes through and they break up, then they are cooked. How long they take to cook depends on the variety of potato. Some "roasters" only take 5 minutes whereas salad potatoes sometimes need a quarter of an hour. Just prod at regular intervals until they are cooked through. Put a sieve in the sink and drain the potatoes into it. Watch out again for the steam, and use oven gloves. You can now serve the potatoes or prepare them further.

Some people prefer to cook the potatoes in their skins and then peel them. This means that starch and other ingredients are preserved inside the potato. The method described above means that some starch is washed out, which can be an advantage during the elimination diet.

Cook with confidence!

Cooking is not sorcery! You don't have to be a Michelin star chef. It's quite enough if you are capable of preparing a simple, healthy, tasty meal for yourself. It is well known that Rome wasn't built in a day so don't give up if you have a couple of disasters. You learn by your mistakes, especially in the kitchen. Don't start your cooking career with difficult dishes. Instead, tread carefully at the start and don't try to run before you can walk.

12. RECIPES

Our recipes are all suitable for the fructose intolerance elimination diet. We have also indicated whether the food is low in histamine or not. But when you are doing the histamine intolerance elimination diet then you also have to be very careful about how you store products. We often cook with dairy products. If you have lactose intolerance then substitute lactose-free dairy products or use alternatives like rice milk, almond milk or soy products. These alternatives are - if no sugar or sugar substitues are added - suitable for the fructose intolerance elimination diet too.

Culinary tip: Get some fresh herbs into your kitchen. Oregano, basil, chives or sage have a place in every kitchen. Herbs give more taste to your food which means you need less salt. For ethical reasons, we decided not to use tuna recipes. If you eat other kinds of fish, please keep an eye out for sustainable fishing. Please also pay attention to quality in whatever products you use. Organic, free-range eggs (no cage) or local organically farmed meat is not just healthier but also of better quality. Organically and locally grown paprika is more natural than vegetables from afar with a big carbon footprint. Of course, these are decisions you must take yourself, but we have paid attention to these factors in designing our recipes and hope that many others share our opinion in this matter.

Unless otherwise indicated, these recipes are always designed for 2 people.

13. BASIC RECIPES

Pancakes, crépes & co.

low fructose, lactose free (with rice milk), low histamine

For 4-8 pancakes (depending on the size of the pan)
7oz (200g) plain flour
2 eggs
1 ²/₃ cups (400 ml) milk, or rice milk without added sugar
1 pinch of salt

> When making batter or cakes, mix wet ingredients together in one bowl, the dry ingredients together in a larger one, then mix the two together. That way you are less likely to get lumps.

Mix the flour, salt, eggs and milk in a bowl with a whisk or a hand blender until you have a fairly runny batter. If you have time and unless you have histamine intolerance, let it rest for half an hour in the refrigerator.

Heat just a little oil in the non-stick frying pan and add a ladle-full of batter, tipping the pan so that it thinly covers the whole of the surface. Let it cook for about a minute, then shake gently. The pancake should come loose. At this point use a pallet knife (if you have one) or a flat turner to flip it over. (Pancake tossing is an art that needs a lot of practice, so be modest at first.) Let the other side brown. Tip onto a warmed plate (which you can also keep in the oven on minimum heat while you cook the rest). Repeat until you have used up all the batter, creating a 'pancake tower'. Add a minimal quantity of oil to the pan for each new pancake, and don't let the pan get too hot! Even for experienced cooks, the first pancake is often a bit of a mess, but the rest come out better.

By varying the amount of liquid you add, you can make your batter thicker or thinner. Thicker batter is usually used for smaller, heavier pancakes, made in a smaller pan.

Tapioka crêpes

low fructose, lactose free, low histamine, gluten free
For 4-8 crêpes (depending on size of pan)

7oz (200 g) Tapioca starch
5-7 tbsp (75-105 ml) of water

The basic idea of this recipe is to dampen the tapioca starch but not to prepare it as a liquid.

Put the tapioca starch into a large bowl.
Add a couple of tablespoons of water and knead it thoroughly. Add another tablespoon and knead again. When you squeeze the tapioca starch it should stick together and not run through your fingers. If the tapioca starch starts to run then you have used too much water. Just add more starch until it becomes solid again.
Now rub the starch through a sieve into another bowl. It should look like snow!

Heat a non-stick frying pan thoroughly and then take it off the heat and place on a heat-proof surface. Rub the tapioca through the sieve again, into the pan to give a 2mm – 3mm layer. (The reason for taking the pan off the stove is that if the tapioca starch lands outside the pan on the hot stove it is incredibly difficult to clean!) Put the pan back on the stove at medium heat and bake the
crêpes for 2 to 3 minutes on each side.

These crêpes can be served with all kinds of fillings, just like ordinary crêpes or pancakes, of course taking account of the individual food intolerance or personal tolerance levels. Those fillings can include whipped cream and desiccated coconut, freshly grated coconut or, for something savoury, with smoked salmon and cottage cheese.

Tapioca crêpes are classic Brazilian street food, prepared fresh by street vendors on little stoves at the side of the road.

SALAD DRESSING: SOY-MUSTARD DRESSING

low fructose, lactose free

½ CUP (100ML) OF WATER
3 TBSP APPLE OR HERB-FLAVOURED VINEGAR
½ TSP ESTRAGON OR OTHER MILD MUSTARD (SUCH AS DIJON)
1 DASH OF SOY SAUCE
1 PINCH OF DRIED OR SMALL HANDFUL OF FRESH SALAD HERBS
1 PINCH OF SALT
1 PINCH OF GROUND PEPPER
1 TBSP OLIVE OIL
½ TSP GLUCOSE

Put all the ingredients in a bowl and beat with a whisk to form an emulsion. Before pouring it over the salad, taste and season, and give it another quick whisk. Another way of preparing it is to put all the ingredients in a clean, empty jam jar, put the lid on tight and then shake hard until an emulsion is formed.

CHIMICHURRI SAUCE

Low fructose, lactose free, low histamine, gluten free
This recipe should only be tried after the first two weeks of the elimination diet.

0.8OZ (25G) CHOPPED FLAT-LEAF PARSLEY
0.3-0.5OZ (10-15G) CHOPPED FRESH CORIANDER
1 GARLIC CLOVE, CHOPPED FINE OR PRESSED
5 TBSP (75ML) OLIVE OIL
3 TSP LEMON JUICE (WITH HISTAMINE INTOLERANCE, OMIT AT THE
START AND TEST LATER FOR INDIVIDUAL TOLERANCE)
SALT & PEPPER (OPTIONAL)

Put all the ingredients in a bowl and mix well. This is a recipe you can easily adapt according to taste. Some prefer a stronger coriander flavour, which simply means increasing the amount of coriander. This sauce, with its South American origins, has many uses. It serves as a sauce for meat dishes, can be spread on bread or used s a pesto to mix with pasta or noodles.

Mayonnaise

low fructose, lactose free, gluten free (read ingredients of mustard!)

1 EGG YOLK (USE FRESH EGGS!)
1 SMALL PINCH OF SALT
1 SMALL PINCH OF PEPPER
1 TSP ESTRAGON OR OTHER MILD MUSTARD
ABOUT ½ CUP (100ML) VEGETABLE OIL (NOT OLIVE OIL)

TIP

You must add the oil very slowly and in small amounts, otherwise the mayonnaise will be too runny or may curdle.

Put the egg yolk in a deep bowl. Add the salt and mustard. Give it a short blast with a hand-mixer, or use a whisk if you want to develop your arm and wrist muscles. Keep on whisking while you add the oil **very slowly** until you have an even mixture. If the mayonnaise is too stiff then you can add one to two teaspoons of water and whisk again. The prepared mayonnaise can be kept for one to two days in the refrigerator.

14. BREAKFAST

PANCAKES WITH RICE SYRUP

low fructose, lactose free (with rice milk), low histamine

1 PANCAKE – SEE BASIC RECIPE ON PAGE 83

RICE SYRUP (AVAILABLE FROM THE HEALTH FOOD STORE)

OPTIONAL: COCONUT FLAKES

This breakfast is quick and easy to make if the pancake has already been made the day before (not in the case of histamine intolerance elimination diet!) The pancakes can be eaten warm or cold with some rice syrup. Sprinkle with coconut flakes (optional).

After the elimination diet you can certainly add some of the fruit you tolerate, cut up fine.

OAT-CORN MUESLI

Low fructose, low histamine

1 SMALL TUB OF NATURAL YOGHURT

5 TBSP PORRIDGE OATS

10 TBSP UNSWEETENED CORNFLAKES (MOSTLY ONLY AVAILABLE IN HEALTH FOOD STORES)

4 TSP GLUCOSE OR A COUPLE OF DASHES OF LIQUID STEVIA

JUICE OF HALF A LEMON (OPTIONAL; NOT DURING HISTAMINE INTOLERANCE ELIMINATION DIET)

Mix the yoghurt and the oats and let it stand for about 10 minutes. Add the other ingredients and mix well. Those who are very sensitive can first cook the porridge oats briefly in water, drain and allow to cool. Following the elimination diet, the muesli can be enhanced with some of the fruit you can tolerate.

Avocado spread

low fructose, lactose free, gluten free

1 RIPE AVOCADO
2 TBSP LIME JUICE
PINCH OF SALT, PEPPER

Cut the avocado open down the middle lengthways and remove the stone. Use a spoon to scoop out the flesh, into a small bowl. Add the lime juice, salt and pepper. Squash with a fork until it forms a cream. This cream tastes excellent spread on bread and crackers. It can also be used as a dip for potatoes or crisps.

The spread can also be refined with fresh herbs. Chives are especially suited. The spread should not be kept for long because it quickly discolours brown.

Cheese and ham open sandwich

Low fructose, lactose free

Home-made bread with lactose-free cheese and ham. If you are lactose intolerant then cheeses such as mature Gouda, Tilsiter or camembert should be suitable. (Look for 'Carbohydrates 0,0g' on the packaging; this means the cheese is lactose free.) With ham you have to look out for additives. Ham carved off the bone is mostly additive-free. Reformed or cured ham or sliced sausage is not appropriate because they almost all contain additives such as honey or one of the many types of sugar. If it's all a bit boring, then a bit of mustard on the bread should do no harm. Mustard mostly contains sugars but the quantity you spread on bread is so small that the sugar is negligible.

LIPTAUER SPREAD

low fructose, gluten free (read ingredients of mustard!)

7OZ (200G) QUARK / COTTAGE CHEESE / CURD CHEESE
(ALSO AVAILABLE LACTOSE FREE)
A HANDFUL OF FRESH CHOPPED CHIVES
2 SMALL OR ONE LARGE PICKLED GHERKINS
2 TSP ESTRAGON OR OTHER MILD MUSTARD
½ TSP CUMIN SEEDS
2 TSP GROUND PAPRIKA
SALT, PEPPER

Crush the cumin seeds a little with a pestle and mortar. Break up the quark or cottage cheese with a fork and stir it. Dice the chives, cumin seeds and pickled gherkin finely and add. Stir in the ground paprika and the mustard. Add salt and pepper to taste. Liptauer tastes best when it has rested in the refrigerator for an hour or two. Spread the liptauer on half a bread roll, decorate with more chives. If you want a taste of spring, decorate with fresh daisies or nasturtiums. During the test period fresh radishes are the perfect accompaniment.

A "quick cornbread" is the perfect partner for liptauer spread. For the recipe, see "Baking your own bread" below.

Tipp: Cumin

Cumin works to counter bloating or flatulence and is thus a highly recommended spice for use in the first phase of the elimination diet.

15. MID-DAY OR EVENING MEAL

FRIED RICE – KHAO PAD

low fructose, lactose free, low histamine, gluten free
Ideal for the start of the elimination diet

8.8oz (250g) FRESHLY COOKED WHITE RICE

2 EGGS

OPTIONAL EXTRAS: *FRESH BEAN SPROUTS, COURGETTES, GREEN
BELL PEPPER, PEAS, DICED AND FRESHLY COOKED CHICKEN, …*

The following recipe is in fact one of the basic recipes that can be varied after the end of the elimination diet. It is also an excellent recipe to use to test certain types of vegetable for your individual tolerance level. This means that after the elimination diet you can add vegetables, one at a time. If you tolerate that meal well then you can add another type of vegetable next time. Suitable vegetables include courgettes, green bell pepper, mushrooms or peas. During the first phase of the elimination diet you should not add any vegetables at all. That means you are left with fried rice and egg. Those who are not vegetarian can add a little diced, cooked chicken, even during the elimination diet. But you should make sure that the chicken is freshly cooked, and well cooked through. Do not use ready made chicken!

First cook the rice, as shown in "Preparation of certain basic foods" on page 78, and set it aside.

Dice the vegetables finely and fry very briefly in a hot pan. Transfer to a plate and put aside.

Heat a little oil in the pan and break the egg into it. (If you are nervous about that and don't want a mouthful of shell, then break the egg into a cup first before you pour it into the pan.) Stir the egg well with a wooden spoon. When the egg has solidified, add the rice, mix well, and let it fry a little. Keep on stirring until the rice colours slightly.

Add the vegetables and fry just a little longer to heat it all through.

Add salt and pepper to taste. Those who want to can add a little soy sauce (but pay attention to the list of ingredients).

You can see that fried rice is a dish you can adapt in many ways. In its simplest form (rice with egg, rice with egg and chicken) it is **ideal for the elimination diet in fructose intolerance** cases. In its more complex form (rice, egg and vegetables) it is ideal for the test period when you are trying to find out where your individual tolerance lies. In addition, you can ideally adapt this dish for people who do not have intolerances. This means you can feed the whole family and do not have to cook twice!

In cases of histamine intolerance you can omit the egg and try variations on rice, chicken and fresh vegetables. Egg actually no longer works as an histamine releaser once it is cooked. The best course here is to test individually.

PORK FILET WITH SAGE AND FRIED COURGETTES
low fructose, lactose free, gluten free

21.1oz (600g) pork filet
About 10 large, fresh sage leaves
Vegetable oil
Salt & pepper

For the sauce:
7 tbsp (100ml) lactose-free cream
7 tbsp (100ml) water
1-2 tsp corn starch
2 large courgettes (preferably straight)

3.5oz (100g) Rice

Pre-heat the oven to 350°F (170°C) and cook the rice.

Meanwhile, using a sharp knife, cut little pockets into the side of the pork filet at about 2 inches (5 cm) intervals. Wash the sage leaves and then pack into the pockets as flat as possible. Because fresh sage is strong, position the leaves side by side rather than on top of one another. Season the filet all over with salt and pepper.

Wash the courgettes and slice them lengthways into strips about 0.2 inches (½ cm) thick.

Put a little oil in a frying pan, let it get fairly hot, then sear the pork filet on all sides for 1 to 2 minutes until the surface is brown. Browning improves the taste and gives a tasty gravy. Now transfer the pork filet to a roasting tin and give it around 15 minutes on a middle shelf in the pre-heated oven.

As soon as you have got the meat in the oven, turn the heat under the frying pan down to medium and put the courgettes in the hot juices. Brown on both sides. If the pan is too small to take all the courgettes, fry them in batches and keep warm on a heat-proof plate in the oven with the filet.

As soon as the last of the courgettes are fried, make the gravy by adding the water (or vegetable stock) and carefully loosen any bits from the surface of the pan. Take care to use a suitable wooden or plastic scraper so as not to damage the surface of a none-stick pan. Add the cream and bring gently to the boil. Put the corn starch into a glas, add very little water and stir until dissolved. Add this mixture to thicken, stirring all the time. Cook briefly. Season to taste with salt and pepper.

If desired, you can add one or two teaspoons of Chimichurri (see "Chimichurri Sauce" on page 85) to the gravy to give it that extra kick.

Carve the pork filet into portions and serve immediately with the rice, courgettes and gravy.

POLENTA PIZZA STYLE

low fructose, lactose free, low histamine (without the canned sweet corn or mushrooms), gluten free

SUFFICIENT POLENTA FOR 4 (SEE PACKET)
LACTOSE FREE, GRATED CHEESE (SUCH AS GOUDA)
BASIL, THYME, SALT PEPPER
OPTIONAL: MUSHROOMS AND CANNED SWEET CORN

FOR ALL OTHER GUESTS WHO ARE NOT ON THE ELIMINATION DIET
TOMATO SAUCE (PIZZA SAUCE) – NOT TOO RUNNY
ONIONS, BELL PEPPER, SALAMI, ...
IN PRINCIPLE, EVERYTHING YOU CAN PUT ON A PIZZA!

Line a baking tray with greaseproof paper.

Prepare the polenta according to the instructions on the pack, but with a little more water so that it is not as stiff as usual. Roll or press it onto the baking tray to a thickness of about 0.4 inches (1 cm) and let it cool. The polenta will then solidify.

Pre-heat the oven to around 390°F (200°C). As soon as the polenta is cool, prepare like a normal pizza. For instance, cover a quarter of it, reserved for those on the fructose diet, just with cheese and sweet corn. On the rest, first spread with pizza sauce, then decorate with the cheese and other ingredients. Place in the oven for just long enough to let the cheese brown. Remove, and sprinkle with freshly chopped herbs.

CHICKEN FILET SCHNITZEL WITH PARSLEY POTATOES

low fructose, lactose free, low histamine, gluten free

2 CHICKEN FILET SCHNITZELS (FLATTENED)
4 LARGE WAXY (SALAD) POTATOES
FRESH PARSLEY, VEGETABLE OIL, SALT, PEPPER

Boil the potatoes whole, and while they are cooking sear the meat on both sides in a little oil until slightly brown. Only season with salt after searing. Wash and then chop the parsley. When the potatoes are just cooked, drain them and cut them into 1 inch (2 cm) cubes (You can also cut them up before cooking them). Gently heat a little oil in a frying pan, add the potatoes and the parsley. Stir until the parsley coats the potatoes. Season with salt and pepper. Serve, preferably with a green salad.

> To flatten schnitzels, put the fillets one by one into a plastic freezer bag and hit with a rolling pin, a meat hammer or a cold iron (just get inventive!) until they are flat and thin.

FISH SALAD
low fructose, lactose free, gluten free

1 SMALL CUCUMBER
HALF A HEAD OF LETTUCE
2 SMOKED TROUT FILETS
2 PICKLED GHERKINS
2 TBSP VINEGAR
1 TSP SALAD OIL (OLIVE OIL)
½ TSP SUGAR OR 2 DROPS OF LIQUID STEVIA
CHIVES, DILL, SALT, PEPPER

OPTIONAL: RED BELL PEPPER

Peel and dice the cucumber. Wash the lettuce, as well as the bell pepper, and dice. Pick any bones out of the trout filets and also dice. Mix together in a large salad bowl. Season with salt and pepper.

Dice the herbs and the pickled gherkin finely and put in a small bowl. Add the oil and vinegar and about $^2/_3$ cups (150ml) water. Add the sugar (or stevia) and mix until the sugar dissolves. Season to taste and pour over the salad. Toss well and serve. During the initial phase of the elimination diet you can use less vinegar and omit the sugar. During the test phase you can easily use this amount of sugar.

Some simply prefer this dressing without the water and sugar. In that case whisk the oil and vinegar to an emulsion (or use the jam jar trick; see "Salad dressing: soy-mustard dressing" on page 85), then add the herbs, pickled gherkin and seasoning to taste.

ROOT VEGETABLE RÖSTI WITH SMOKED SALMON

low fructose, lactose free, gluten free
Only suitable towards the end of the elimination diet!

> *0.8OZ (25G) VEGETABLE MARGARINE*
> *4 ¼ CUPS (1-1,5L) VEGETABLE STOCK OR SOUP (KEEP A CLOSE*
> *EYE ON THE INGREDIENTS OF READY-MADE SOUP OR STOCK!)*
> *1 MEDIUM SIZE SWEET POTATO*
> *1 LARGE POTATO (WAXY IF POSSIBLE)*
> *½ SMALL SWEDE OR TURNIP*
> *1 SMALL PARSNIP*
> *¼ TSP GROUND NUTMEG*
> *8.8OZ (250G) SMOKED SALMON (OR OTHER SMOKED FISH)*
>
> *OPTIONAL: 1 SMALL TUB OF (LACTOSE-FREE) SOURED CREAM*

Pre-heat the oven to 390°F (200°C).
Line two baking trays with greaseproof paper and grease these with lactose-free margarine.

Bring the vegetable soup or stock gently just to the boil in a large pan.

Meanwhile peal the vegetables and slice around 1 inch (2 cm) thick. Add the vegetables to the soup and blanche (partially cook) them for about 4 minutes. Then drain off the soup or stock (keeping the stock for other use) and let the vegetables cool off.

Grate the vegetables into a large bowl. Add the rest of the margarine and the ground nutmeg and mix well by hand. Divide the "dough" into 12 portions and roll into balls. Position the balls on the baking trays and squash them flat. Put the rösti in the oven and bake for 15 – 20 minutes or until they are golden brown and crispy. Cut the smoked salmon into small pieces

To serve, place three of the baked, hot rösti on each plate, scatter the smoked salmon on top and serve with soured cream on the side (optional).

FRIED TURKEY FILET WITH GINGER SPINACH

low fructose, lactose free, gluten free

> *2 TURKEY (OR CHICKEN) FILETS*
> *17.6OZ (500G) FRESH SPINACH*
> *1 CUP RICE*
> *FRESH GINGER – ABOUT 2 INCHES*
>
> *CHIVES, SALT, PEPPER, OIL*

Cook rice as described in "Preparation of certain basic foods" on page 78.

Peel and chop the ginger very fine. Wash the spinach briefly and cook in a deep pan with as little water as possible – just enough to cover the bottom of the pan. Stir in the ginger and cook until the spinach shrinks – just one or two minutes - then take it off the heat otherwise it will stick to the pan or the ginger will burn.

Meanwhile cut the turkey filets in the length into strips and sear them in a little oil in a hot pan until brown. Season well.

Serve sprinkled with fresh chives.

ASPARAGUS WITH BOILED HAM AND LEMON

low fructose, lactose free, low histamine (with boiled ham), gluten free (control ham ingredients!)

This is an ideal recipe for the test period or the last days of the elimination diet.

1-2 TBSP VEGETABLE OIL
20 GREEN ASPARAGUS STALKS
8 SLICES OF HAM (PARMA HAM IS PARTICULARLY SUITABLE, BUT
FOR LOW HISTAMINE STICK WITH COOKED HAM)
7 TBSP (100ML) WATER
1 LEMON

Wash the asparagus well and snap off the "woody" end. It is fairly easy to tell where the woody end starts because you can snap it off quite easily at this point.

Tear the ham into pieces roughly 2cm or an inch square. Fry these for about 2 minutes in a large frying pan at medium heat. Then add the whole asparagus stalks and fry, turning frequently, for a further two minutes. Now add the water, cover with a lid and simmer for a further two minutes until the asparagus is cooked. (That's when a fork goes through the thick end with ease.) If you don't have a lid to fit the frying pan, then transfer to another pan that does.

Tip
Add as little water as possible – just enough for the asparagus to be able to steam once the lid is on the pan.

When you have reached the test phase you can also add some finely sliced garlic towards the end.

Serve the asparagus with the other ingredients, but without the liquid from the pan. Squeeze a little lemon juice over it (except for those on the histamine elimination diet).

About asparagus:
Asparagus contains high levels of vitamins A and E but is low in vitamin

C and biotin. Asparagus should always be served with a little fat (oil or butter) to enable the vitamin E to be absorbed. Asparagus contains a relatively high amount of roughage which encourages healthy digestion. However, it should only be used in the last weeks of the elimination diet.

CHICKEN SALAD

low fructose, lactose free, low histamine (use skinless chicken breast), gluten free

2 CUPS (500ML) WATER
SOUP VEGETABLES (CARROT, ONION, SWEDE AND OTHER ROOT VEGETABLES IN SEASON)
1 BAY LEAF
2 FRESH CHICKEN BREASTS
ABOUT 7OZ (200G) OF LETTUCE (A MIXED LEAF SALAD IS ALSO FINE)

FOR THE MARINADE:
4-5 TBSP OLIVE OIL
½ LEMON
SALT & PEPPER
OPTIONAL FRESH PARSLEY FOR GARNISH

Wash the soup vegetables, peel where necessary, and cut into cubes about ½ inch (1cm) square. Place in a large pan together with the chicken breasts, two teaspoons of salt, some pepper and the bay leaf. Cover with cold water, about 2 inches (5cm) above the level of the contents. Cover and bring to the boil, then lower the heat between medium and low so that the contents can simmer gently for around an hour.

After an hour, take out the chicken, let it cool a little, and slice it into thin strips.

Wash the salad ingredients and put them in a bowl. In a smaller bowl, mix the ingredients for the marinade thoroughly and pour them over the salad. Add the cooked strips of chicken. Garnish with small pieces of parsley if desired.

The remaining stock can be passed through a sieve and stored for a few days in the refrigerator (except in histamine intolerance cases) so that it can be used as a basis for other dishes. You can eat the vegetables themselves, and they are also good to serve to non-intolerant family members as ingredients of a soup or just as a vegetable dish.

SIMPLE ROAST BEEF

low fructose, lactose free
Serves 6-8!

Cooking timings:
Rare: 20 minutes per 16 oz (450g) plus 20 minutes
Medium: 25 minutes per 16 oz (450g) plus 25 minutes
Well done: 30 minutes per 16 oz (450g) plus 30 minutes

4LB (1,8KG) TENDERLOIN OR OTHER ROASTING JOINT
3 TBSP ENGLISH MUSTARD
SALT AND FRESHLY GROUND PEPPER
7/8 CUP (200ML) HOT BEEF STOCK

Pre-heat the oven to 350-370°F (170-190°C).

Place the roast on a chopping board. Rub in the salt, pepper and mustard to cover all the surfaces.

Lay the meat in a roasting tin with any fat layer uppermost and place in the pre-heated oven. If the fat gets too brown during the cooking time then cover the roast with aluminium foil to prevent it from burning. Baste occasionally with its own juices, or sprinkle with a little water.

At the end of the cooking time remove the roast from the oven, transfer to a deep plate and cover with aluminium foil. Let it rest for 15 to 20 minutes. This 'relaxes' the meat and makes it more tender. Put the roasting tin on the stove on medium heat and add some stock. Use a wooden spoon to loosen any meat scraps in the tin to make a gravy. Simmer down for about five minutes.

Carve the beef into thin slices and pour on a little of the hot gravy (which you could also serve separately). Roast beef goes well with either parsley potatoes or rice as well as leaf salad.

TIROLER GRÖSTL (TYROLEAN STYLE POTATOES)

low fructose, lactose free, low histamine (without the meat), gluten free

WAXY OR SALAD POTATOES FOR 2
7OZ (200G) BACON OR COOKED BEEF
2 EGGS
SALT, PEPPER, FRESH CHIVES

OPTIONAL INGREDIENTS:
ONIONS AND GARLIC (AFTER THE ELIMINATION DIET), MUSH-
ROOMS (DURING THE TEST PERIOD)

Cook the potatoes in their skins, peel and allow to cool, then cut in slices. Cut the meat into small slices or the bacon into cubes. Slice and dice the onions and garlic and cook gently at low heat in a little oil. When the onions start to brown then add the meat or bacon and turn up the heat. Then add to potatoes and cook until the potatoes start to brown. Add salt and pepper to taste and transfer onto a plate.
Break the eggs into the hot pan to make fried eggs (sunny side up). Place these on top of the Gröstl and sprinkle with fresh chopped chives.

Omit the onions during the elimination diet. Those who don't want to eat meat can leave this out and add a couple of chopped mushrooms instead. Do not add salt to mushrooms during cooking. This draws the water out of them and would dampen the Gröstl, making it mushy. Only add salt, if at all, after serving.

Cucumber Makis

low fructose, lactose free, gluten free
You need a flexible bamboo mat to make this dish!

HIT and nori leaves

We have very little information or records of experience about the toler-ance of nori leaves in cases of histamine intolerance. It is a good idea to test this individually after the end of the elimination diet. They do, how-ever, appear to be well tolerated. You can use water instead of vinegar and should omit the soy sauce and wasabi.

½ cucumber, peeled and with the seeds removed
2 nori leaves (dried kelp)
7oz (200g) uncooked Sushi rice
A little rice vinegar

Optional (pay attention to list of ingredients) :
Soy sauce, wasabi powder or paste, preserved ginger
(during test phase)

Other optional ingredients: smoked salmon, avocado,
smoked trout

Prepare the sushi rice according to the instructions on the pack and allow to cool.

Slice the cucumber (and other optional ingredients) into strips about 0.2 inches (½ cm) thick.

Lay the nori, shiny side up, on the bamboo mat and spread the rice on it about 0.2 inches (½cm) thick. Press the rice down and sprinkle with a little rice vinegar. Leave 2-3cm (about an inch) of the nori leaf uncovered at one end. Lay the cucum-ber strips and other ingredients side by side on top of the other end, then use the flexible mat to roll it up. Wet the free end of the nori with rice vinegar and stick it to the rest to make a roll. This may all need a bit of practice. (If in doubt visit a sushi bar and watch how they make the maki.)

Lay the roll on a chopping board and cut into bite-size slices, using a very sharp knife.

Dip the makis in soy sauce and eat. After the test phase you can add strong wasabi to the soy sauce. Watch out if you are using ready-made products because they often contain lactose or gluten. An Asian food store has wasabi powder that you can just mix with water.

Instead of cucumber you can use other vegetables or smoked trout or salmon. Get creative!

CHICKEN AND VEGETABLES BRAISED IN THE OVEN
low fructose (only use mushrooms during the test phase), lactose free, gluten free, low histamine (use skinned chicken drumsticks, legs or thighs).
This is also suitable for the initial days of the elimination diet (see recipe).

WAXY OR SALAD POTATOES FOR 4
4-6 CHICKEN JOINTS (DRUMSTICK, LEG OR THIGH)
2-3 GARLIC CLOVES
1 ONION
1 COURGETTE
4-6 CARROTS
7OZ (200G) FRESH MUSHROOMS
1 BELL PEPPER
SALT, PEPPER, GROUND PAPRIKA

ALUMINUM FOIL

Pre-heat the oven to 400°F (200°C) – bottom and upper heat.

Wash and halve the mushrooms, chop the vegetables into large pieces and place in a casserole. Add a little oil, salt, ground paprika and pepper and mix well. Meanwhile rub salt and ground paprika into the chicken pieces.

Add the chicken joints, skin side up if the skin is still on, on top of the vegetables. Place the casserole on the middle shelf in the pre-heated oven and allow to cook for 30 minutes.

If there is no moisture from the mushrooms in the bottom of the dish then add sufficient water or vegetable stock to cover the bottom of the dish. Baste the joints with the cooking liquid from the casserole every 10 minutes throughout the cooking time.

If you are using an US oven that only has bottom heat: After 30 minutes cover the casserole with aluminium foil, change setting to "broil" and broil for 15 minutes.

The chicken pieces should be cooked through after 30-45 minutes. (Never eat under-cooked chicken!)

> The dish is great, because it is ideal for the family when not everyone is on an elimination diet. Those on the elimination diet only get chicken and potatoes while the rest can enjoy the vegetables. If you are in the test phase then you can test the different vegetables – one at a time.

MACARONI AND CHEESE

low fructose
Due to its high fat content, this recipe should only be cooked at the earliest at the end of the elimination diet or during the test phase or during the permanent diet.

2 CUPS (200G) MACARONI, UNCOOKED
3 CUPS (700ML) MILK
1 CUP (150G) GRATED EDAM CHEESE (OR SOME OTHER GRATED
CHEESE SUCH AS CHEDDAR OR GOUDA)
1/3 CUP (30G) GRATED PARMESAN CHEESE
2 TBLS OLIVE OIL
SALT, PEPPER, PAPRIKA

Pre-heat oven to 350°F (170°C).

Put the oil in a small casserole and stir in the uncooked macaroni. Add salt, pepper and paprika and stir well. Add the cheese over the top and gently pour the milk over everything. Do not stir and bake for approximately 15 minutes. Reduce heat to 300°F (130°C) and bake for another 15 minutes.

SALMON WITH POLENTA AND SALAD

low fructose, lactose free

8.8oz (250g) frozen wild salmon filet (or other frozen filleted white fish)
5.2oz (150g) polenta
green leaf salad
Soy sauce, soup powder, salt (pay attention to ingredients list for soy sauce and soup powder)

Dressing: The soy-mustard dressing from page 85 is the perfect match.

Prepare the polenta according to the instructions on the pack. The time it takes to prepare depends on how finely it is ground or what type it is. We recommend an 'instant' or fast-cooking polenta.

For these, you boil up the polenta from the pack briefly in water, according to instructions, and then set it aside to soak through. Pour the polenta into a square or rectangular dish and let it cool. It will set firm. You can also buy ready-made polenta, but you must then pay close attention to the ingredients list. Once the polenta has cooled and set, slice into finger-width slices.

Cover the bottom of a broad-based pan with about 1cm (½ inch) of water. Add the powdered soup, salt and a little soy sauce and heat, stirring, until you have a tasty stock. Lay the wild salmon filets in the stock. Do not defrost. Bring back to the boil and simmer, covered, on low heat for about 10 minutes.

In the meantime wash the salad and prepare the salad dressing.

Heat a little oil in a frying pan and fry the polenta slices for about 2 minutes on each side. Extract the fish carefully from the pan, trying not to let it break apart. Serve.

For those in the family who are not affected by the elimination diet you can prepare a separate salad with extras such as onions or strips of raw carrot.

SPINACH AND SALMON DISH

low fructose, lactose free, gluten free (inspect ingredients list!)
This is an ideal recipe for the test period.

10.5OZ (300G) BONELESS SALMON FILET

8.8OZ (250G) FROZEN LEAF SPINACH

2 CLOVES OF GARLIC

1 RED BELL PEPPER

½ CUP (120ML) OF WATER MIXED WITH TWO TBSP VINEGAR OR WHITE WINE

1 ¼ CUPS (300ML) UNSWEETENED SOY MILK OR RICE MILK

3 TSP RED GROUND PAPRIKA

SALT, PEPPER

OPTIONAL INGREDIENTS: ONIONS (AFTER THE ELIMINATION PHASE), LEMON WEDGES.

RICE AS SIDE DISH

Rinse the salmon then pat it dry with kitchen paper and cut into middle-sized cubes. Prepare the spinach according to instructions, drain in a sieve and squeeze the excess liquid out of it. Wash the bell pepper, discard the seeds and cut into stripes. Chop the garlic.

Tip

The skin comes off the garlic cloves more easily if you hit – but don´ t squash – them first with a meat hammer or a knife handle.)

Heat a little oil in a frying pan and fry the salmon briefly. Transfer to a plate and season lightly with salt and pepper. Using the same pan, lightly fry the paprika, garlic (and onions), sprinkle with the ground paprika, stir once and add the wine or other liquid immediately. Stir again, and add the soy or rice milk. As soon as it comes back to the boil add the cooked spinach and let the whole cook for about five minutes on a low flame. Add the cooked salmon, stir once gently, take it off the heat and leave it aside for a couple of minutes for the flavours to penetrate the fish. Serve with rice, and enjoy! Those who want can also have lemon wedges.

Tip

If the sauce is too thin then you can mix a teaspoon of corn starch with as little water as possible, stir into the sauce and bring back to the boil. It should thicken. Do this after you add the cooked spinach but before you add the cooked fish.

COUSCOUS BURGERS

low fructose, lactose free
This recipe is suitable for the first week of the elimination diet

8 TBSP COUSCOUS
1 TBSP DURUM WHEAT FLOUR
2 TBSP PLAIN FLOUR
3 EGG YOLKS
1 ¼ CUPS (300ML) BOILING WATER
ITALIAN HERBS (DRIED), SALT, PEPPER

OPTIONAL: JUICE OF ¼ LIME

Take a large bowl, add the couscous and durum wheat flour and mix with the boiling water. Leave it to stand until the couscous has absorbed it and is soft and still warm to the touch.

Mix in egg yolks, salt and pepper to taste, lime juice, and herbs. If it is too liquid then add some more flour.

Heat several tablespoons of oil in a pan. Use a large spoon or your hands to form 'burgers' from the mixture and fry them on both sides. If you want a crust, then coat them in fine dry breadcrumbs (shop-bought) before frying. When the burgers are golden brown take them out and put them on kitchen paper to drain off excess fat.

These can be accompanied for those not on the elimination diet by a green salad, some pumpkin seed oil and parmesan cheese.

Optional: after the elimination phase, add some bacon croutons and vegetables such as canned sweet corn or grated courgette to the dough.

SPINACH PANCAKE
low fructose, lactose free

4 PANCAKES – SEE BASIC PANCAKE RECIPE ON PAGE 83
15.8OZ (450G) FROZEN CHOPPED YOUNG SPINACH
2 TBSP FLOUR
SOME LACTOSE FREE MILK OR UNSWEETENED SOY OR RICE MILK
SALT, PEPPER
¼ JUICE OF ONE LIME

Heat 2 tbsp of oil in a pan, add the flour, stir until oil is absorbed then add the milk and whisk until it thickens. Add the frozen spinach and cook until it has thawed and is creamy. Season with salt, pepper and lime juice.

Meanwhile cook a pancake (unless you have some prepared). Spread spinach mix on the centre of the pancake and roll it up. Repeat for the number of portions required.

BAKED POTATOES WITH EGG AND COTTAGE CHEESE

low fructose, low histamine, gluten free (inspect ingredients list!)

4 LARGE BAKING POTATOES
SOME BUTTER
4 EGGS
½ LEVEL TEASPOON GROUND CUMIN
UP TO 1.7OZ (50G) BOILED HAM, SLICED THIN
8.8OZ (250G) COTTAGE CHEESE
SALT AND PEPPER

Pre-heat the oven to 390°F (200°C)

Wash to potatoes well until the skins are really clean and wrap in foil. Make sure there are no gaps in the foil otherwise the potatoes will dry out in the oven. Cook in the oven for 1 to 1½ hours depending on the size. The potatoes are cooked if they give when you squeeze them gently. (Wear oven gloves for this!)

About 20 minutes before the potatoes are ready, mix the eggs in a cup with the cumin, salt and pepper. Take a none-stick frying pan, heat a little oil or butter, add the egg and cook on a low heat, stirring all the time with a wooden spoon, until you have fine scrambled eggs. Add the cottage cheese and the chopped ham and heat through.

Cut the baked potatoes down the middle, still in the foil, and pull apart. Fill with the egg and cheese mixture.

Those with histamine intolerance who want to avoid egg whites can hard-boil the 4 eggs, extract the yolk and mix it with the other ingredients. Egg white is only seen as a histamine releaser when it is uncooked, so cooked eggs should be no problem in principle. It is best to test your individual tolerance level.

Spaghetti with Chinese cabbage and bacon

Low fructose, lactose free
A good recipe for testing Chinese cabbage

10.5oz (300G) SPAGHETTI

2 EGGS

7oz (200G) CHINESE CABBAGE

5.2oz (150G) BACON

SALT, PEPPER

OPTIONAL:

BEAN SPROUTS; TO BE ADDED SHORTLY BEFORE THE END OF THE COOKING TIME.

Chinese cabbage tip:

Chinese cabbage, like other cabbages, is harder near the stalk. This part is better for use as a vegetable. The ends of the leaves, without the stalk, are more suitable for use in salads.

Cook the spaghetti (see "Preparation of certain basic foods" on page 78) and drain.

Dice the bacon, cut the Chinese cabbage into strips and wash well with several changes of water. Using a none-stick pan, heat the bacon slowly until the fat starts to melt. Add the Chinese cabbage and stir gently for two to three minutes, then add the spaghetti and heat through; lower the heat a little, pour the eggs over the mixture, and mix well until the eggs have set. Season with salt and pepper. Optionally, you can sprinkle the dish with chopped chives.

Fettucine Alfredo "chicken and broccoli"

low fructose; lactose free (if prepared with lactose free milk, butter and cheese)

5 oz (150G) BROCCOLI DIVIDED INTO FLORETS

4 CHICKEN BREASTS

½ CUP (125ML) CREAM

½ CUP (125ML) MILK

4 OZ (120 G) FETTUCINI PASTA
½ CUP (60G) GRATED PARMESAN OR GRANA PADANO CHEESE
2 TBSP BUTTER
SALT, PEPPER, BASIL, THYME

Cook fettucini according to package instructions or see chapter "Preparation of certain basic foods" on page 78 for help.

Put the broccoli in boiling, salted water for 4 to 5 minutes. Drain and plunge into ice-cold water to retain flavor and color. Meanwhile, cut the chicken into bite sized pieces. Melt the butter in non-stick frying pan and cook the chicken over medium heat until browned. Stir frequently! Add the cream, milk, broccoli, salt, pepper, herbs and the pasta. Stir the mixture well, add the cheese and let it cook on a low heat for 2-3 minutes. Serve the dish with additional cheese and fresh chopped herbs.

> Although "Fettuccine Alfredo" sounds Italian, it is a typical American recipe. The name "Fettuccine Alfredo" is largely unknown in Italy and the rest of Europe.

QUICK CUCUMBER SALAD AND RYE BREAD SNACK

low fructose, lactose free

1 CUCUMBER
2 SLICES OF RYE BREAD
LACTOSE FREE CHEESE, LIPTAUER (RECIPE ON PAGE 89) OR SLICED
HAM FOR BREAD TOPPING
SOY SAUCE, VINEGAR, OLIVE OIL, SALT, PEPPER, SALAD-SEASON-
ING HERBS (DRIED OR FROZEN).

OPTIONAL: FRESH SEED SPROUTS (RADISH, CRESS ETC)

Peel the cucumber finely. Halve in the length and chop into bite-sized pieces. Put in a deep bowl and add a little salt and pepper. Dribble on a little soy sauce and a couple of teaspoons of olive oil. Then add the salad seasoning herbs. This salad is very quick to make and is an ideal accompaniment to an evening open sandwich topped with cheese. You can make one with Camembert and one with Gouda, for instance. Those who want can also pep up the taste with a little mustard.

PASTA AI FUNGI
low fructose, lactose free

7OZ (200G) TAGLIATELLI (OR OTHER PASTA)
8.8OZ (250G) FRESH FUNGI (MUSHROOMS OR CHANTERELLES,
CEPES ETC.)
½ AN ONION
1 TBSP OLIVE OIL
½ CUP (100ML) UNSWEETENED RICE MILK
SALT, PEPPER, CHIVES

Cook the pasta according to instructions on package.

Clean the mushrooms or other fungi well.

Chop the onion fine. Fry the onion briefly (until it turns glassy, but not until it browns), add the fungi and a very little salt.

Cook until the fungi start to give off water. Let the fungi cook gently in their own – use a lid if you have one – then add the rice milk and stir well.

Season according to taste with salt and pepper, add the chives and pour the sauce over the cooked pasta.

CHICKEN SHASHLIK

low fructose, lactose free, gluten free
Taste best if cooked on a barbecue grill rather than in the pan

8.8OZ (250G) CHICKEN OR TURKEY
6-8 MUSHROOMS
1 GREEN BELL PEPPER OR COURGETTE
SALT, PEPPER, GROUND PAPRIKA

OPTIONAL FOR THE REST OF THE FAMILY:
BABY SAUSAGES, COCKTAIL TOMATOES, AUBERGINE, ...

Chop everything into bite-sized pieces and arrange alternately on a metal or wooden skewer. If you are using wood then soak them in water first. This will prevent them from burning and make it easier to get the meat off the skewer later.

Season the shashlik and sprinkle with a little oil. Put them on a hot barbecue grill and turn regularly (using oven gloves!) Alternatively, they can be cooked in a pan, also turning regularly.

These can be accompanied by rice or salad.

This is another recipe that can easily be expanded so that people who are not on an elimination diet can join the party. Each person can create their individual shashlik.

Austrian Meat loaf

low fructose, lactose free
Serves around 6

2.2LBS (1KG) MINCED MEAT OF CHOICE
2 STALE BREAD ROLLS (MAKE SURE YOU KNOW THE INGREDIENTS;
BEST ARE ORGANIC KAISER ROLLS)
2 EGGS
3 TBSP ESTRAGON OR OTHER MILD MUSTARD
2-3 TSP SALT
SOME GROUND PEPPER
ABOUT 1.4OZ (40G) OF FRESH PARSLEY
1 TSP GROUND PAPRIKA

Pre-heat the oven to 350°F (170°C).

Chop the parsley. Soak the stale rolls in water until they are wet through. Squeeze as much water out as you can. In a deep bowl, mix the bread, eggs, meat, ground paprika, salt and pepper until you have a kind of dough. You can do this with a fork, but the best way is to get your hands into it. Place this dough in a well-greased bread tin. Bake in the oven for an hour.

During the test period you can pep up the meat loaf by adding some diced pickled gherkin or bell pepper.

This can be served with potatoes, rice or a green salad.

16. BAKING YOUR OWN BREAD

SOUR DOUGH BREAD

low fructose, lactose free

24.6oz (700g) PLAIN BREAD FLOUR
10.5oz (300g) RYE OR SPELT WHOLEMEAL FLOUR
1 SACHET OF QUICK-ACTION DRIED YEAST
1 SACHET OF SOUR DOUGH EXTRACT (TOTAL ROUND 30g, AVAIL-
ABLE IN HEALTH FOOD STORES)
2 TSP SALT
1 TBSP BREAD SPICES (ANISEED, FENNEL, CUMIN....)
3 1/8 CUPS (750ML) TEPID WATER

You can sieve the flour, which might give the bread a finer texture, but it is not absolutely necessary. What is important is to have a large, clean work surface and some flour to hand.

Mix all dry ingredients in a large bowl, add the tepid water and mix well with a wooden spoon, or by hand. Turn it out on the work surface and knead by hand for at least 10 minutes.

If the dough is sticking to you and the work surface sprinkle a little flour on it. The longer you knead, the less it sticks. When you have a good consistency that no longer sticks then put the ball of dough back in the bowl, cover with a kitchen towel and leave to rise for around 2 hours in a warm place. (An airing cupboard, for those of you who still have them, or a spot near the heating is probably the best spot for this.)

Turn the dough out again, divide it in half and knead both sections briefly. (This is known as 'knocking the dough back' and is meant to take out any excess air bubbles). Try to avoid adding too much fresh flour. Form into two loaves, place on a baking tray lined with greaseproof paper, and make two or three slashes in the top of each with a sharp knife. While the oven heats up to 350 °F (170°C) let the dough rise again for 10 to 15 minutes.

Sprinkle the loaves with a little water and bake on the middle shelf. This can take up to 80 minutes, depending on the size of the loaf. Keep an eye on them, and when they start to brown on top test one by picking it up (oven gloves!) and tapping it on the base. If it sounds hollow then it is baked!

When the bread comes out of the oven transfer it to a grid tray and leave it there to cool. You can easily slice a loaf and freeze it so that you can bake a larger batch and defrost whatever you need by the day.

QUICK CORN ROLLS

low fructose, lactose free
makes 16 rolls

17.6 oz (500g) flour
(e.g. 10.5 oz (350g) bread flour, 5.2 oz (150g) spelt
wholemeal)
1 sachet quick-action dried yeast
2 tsp fine sea-salt
1 tsp glucose or sugar (ordinary sugar is best after the
elimination diet)
2 handfuls of various seeds of choice (linseed, sunflower
seed hearts, sesame seed hearts, pumpkin etc.)
1-2 tsp bread spices: fennel, cumin, aniseed etc.
1 cup (250ml) tepid water
¼ cup (50ml) unsweetened rice milk (during the elimina-
tion diet use an extra 50ml of water instead)

You can sieve the flour, which might give the bread a finer texture, but it is not absolutely necessary. What is important is to have a large, clean work surface and some flour to hand.

Mix all the ingredients with a wooden spoon, or by hand, in a large bowl. Turn out onto the work surface and knead by hand for at least 10 minutes. Use a little flour if everything is sticking to the work surface and to your hands. When it has been kneaded thoroughly and has stopped sticking put the dough back in the bowl, cover with a clean tea-towel and leave in a warm spot to rise for at least an hour. It should more or less double in size.

Pre-heat the oven to 350°F (170°C) and line a baking tray with greaseproof paper.

Divide the dough in two. Form each portion into a ball, then squash. Use a knife to divide each of these 'wheels' into eight triangular sections. This is easiest done by dividing each one down the middle, then dividing it again and again. While the oven is heating up position these triangular rolls, well separated, on the baking tray and allow them to rise again for 10 to 20 minutes. Sprinkle with water and bake on the middle shelf of the oven. Bake for around 12 minutes.

Check as for loaves above – the bread sounds hollow if it is baked through. Allow to cool on a grid tray. Again, you can use or freeze as desired.

17.   SNACKS AND SWEET TREATS

Baked bananas with cinnamon and flaked almonds
low fructose, lactose free, gluten free
Suitable for the test period

> *2 BANANAS*
> *1 TBSP LACTOSE FREE BUTTER*
> *4 TSP GLUCOSE*
> *A LITTLE GROUND CINNAMON*
> *0.8OZ (25G) FLAKED ALMONDS*

Toast the almond flakes in a frying pan without any added oil until they brown slightly. Put aside.

Peel the bananas and cut lengthways. Melt a little butter in the pan and fry them on medium heat. While the bananas are browning on one side, sprinkle evenly with the cinnamon and a little glucose. After a couple of minutes check if the bananas are brown on the underside and, if so, turn carefully. Brown the other side.

Turn the bananas out onto a plate and sprinkle with the rest of the glucose and the almond flakes. Done! Those who do not have fructose intolerance can use some honey instead of glucose.

A handful of nuts
for the test phase

Mix some Brazil nuts, hazelnuts and walnuts.
A handful between meals serves to keep hunger at bay and is good for brainpower!

Mayo-Cheese rolls

low fructose, lactose free
This is one to try out during the test phase

1 CUP HOME-MADE MAYONNAISE (SEE BASIC RECIPE ON PAGE 86)
1 CUP GRATED PARMESAN OR GRANA PADANO CHEESE (LACTOSE FREE)
SUGAR-FREE TOAST BREAD (INSPECT LIST OF INGREDIENTS!) OR OTHER WHITE BREAD YOU TOLERATE

Mix the mayonnaise and the parmesan and spread the mixture on a slice of bread. Bake in a pre-heated oven on the middle shelf at 350°F (170°C) until it browns.

Potato crisps / Potato chips

low fructose, lactose free, gluten free

POTATOES
SALT
GROUND PAPRIKA

YOU NEED: WOODEN SKEWERS

A packet of potato chips? What kind of recipe is that? This junk food, however, is generally well tolerated. But keep an eye on the list of ingredients. You are looking for the plain, basic packets of chips with only potatoes, oil and salt as ingredients. These chips are mostly well tolerated. However, because of the high fat content they are only to be enjoyed now and again and in small quantities!

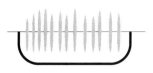 If you want to make your own chips, then you can do this quickly and, especially, without fat. Peel the potatoes and, using a sharp knife or a slicer/grater (watch your fingers!), cut very thin slices. Sprinkle with a little salt and put them on a wooden skewer.

It is most important that they are not touching one another. Find a deep, micro-wave-proof soup plate so that you can suspend the skewer from either edge of it without the potato chips touching the plate below. Cook for 6 to 7 minutes at full power. As soon as they start to brown, stop! If you want, sprinkle with a little ground paprika while still hot. Let them cool, and enjoy!

Tip

Both the chips and the dish will be really hot when they come out of the microwave – so don' t forget the oven gloves!

COCONUT BOMBS

low fructose, low histamine, lactose free, gluten free; (read ingredients lists!)

1 CUP (250ML) COCONUT MILK
0.7OZ (20G) LACTOSE FREE BUTTER
0.7OZ (20G) COCONUT FAT
2.1OU (60G) GLUCOSE
2 TSP RICE SYRUP
4.2OZ (120G) COCONUT FLAKES
PULP OF ONE VANILLA POD

Mix all the ingredients except the coconut flakes in a pan and bring gently to the boil. Allow to simmer until it thickens.

Add most of the coconut flakes and stir well. Let the mixture cool. Then form into little balls by hand and roll in the rest of the coconut flakes.

The best way to store and transport coconut bombs is in little muffin cases.

HONEYDEW MELON WITH GINGER AND COCONUT CREAM

low fructose, lactose free, low histamine
Suitable during the test phase

½ HONEYDEW MELON
1²/₃ CUPS (400ML) COCONUT MILK
0.2 INCH (½ CM) FRESH GINGER
1 TSP GLUCOSE

Leave the coconut milk in the refrigerator for at least three hours, or overnight, before opening the pack or can.

Open the honeydew melon and remove the seeds with a spoon. Cut away the rind. Chop the flesh of the melon into bite-size pieces.

Peel the ginger and grate it finely. Mix the grated ginger and the glucose through the melon pieces and portion these into the serving dishes.

Take the coconut milk out of the refrigerator, being careful not to shake it! Overnight, the coconut milk should have separated from the water. The water has sunk to the bottom, the cream is on top. Open carefully, scoop the cream off the top, transfer to a bowl and stir well. Poar the coconut cream over the melon and serve. Those who prefer can sprinkle the dish with a little more glucose.

Waffels

low fructose, lactose free, low histamine
You need a waffle iron, or a waffle-maker, for this recipe

> *8.8oz (250g) lactose free vegetable margarine*
> *5.2oz (150g) glucose*
> *some drops liquid Stevia (depending on sweetness of brand)*
> *6 eggs*
> *17.6oz (500g) plain flour*
> *1 sachet baking powder (tartar)*
> *15.8oz (450ml) lactose free milk or unsweetened rice milk*

Let the margarine and the milk reach room temperature.

Mix the margarine thoroughly with the glucose, Stevia and the eggs. This is best done with a kitchen machine or a hand mixer. Mix the baking powder into the flour and then stir this, together with the tepid milk, to form a thick batter.

Heat up the waffle iron, insert 2 to 3 tbsp of batter into one half, close and bake.

Rice syrup can be used on waffles as a substitute for honey. After the elimination diet period you can experiment with jams or fruits.

18. APPENDIX

FOOD DIARY

The food diary can help your doctor make a precise diagnosis. You should keep a record for at least 7 days, ideally over a longer period of time. You will need to record all foods and beverages you have eaten. This also includes chewing gum, snacks, medication …

You can download a food diary for free on our website:

 www.food-intolerance-network.com

On the next 2 pages there's another food diary. Feel free to copy it for your personal use!

My Food Diary

Date: _____

Breakfast:

Symptoms:

_____

Snack:

Symptoms:

_____

Mid-day:

Symptoms:

_____

Snack:

Symptoms:

_____

Dinner:

Symptoms:

_____

Night Snack:

Symptoms:

_____

Notes for this day:

My Food Diary

Date: _____

Breakfast:

Symptoms:

Snack:

Symptoms:

Mid-day:

Symptoms:

Snack:

Symptoms:

Dinner:

Symptoms:

Night Snack:

Symptoms:

Notes for this day:

Fructose list alphabetically sorted

The following table lists over 140 foods. The first two columns show pictograms indicating the compatibility during the diet in the first weeks after diagnosis (elimination diet) and during the permanent diet (and test period). The other columns show the fructose, glucose, sorbitol and sucrose levels in g/100g.

Total fructose and glucose are each calculated from the total of the free form plus half of the sucrose.

GLU / FRU indicates the ratio of glucose to fructose. Foods with GLU / FRU=1 or greater than 1 should be compatible. However, since it depends on many other factors, not only on this ratio, the suggested use (pictograms) may vary!

If nothing is specified, this **doesn't** mean that the substance is not present, it means that we have not received any values!

The values in this table are calculated from fructose averages. Because natural fluctuations can happen with most products, these values can only be seen as a rule of thumb.

How to read the table:

ED = elimination diet, first weeks after diagnosis | PD = permanent diet and test period | FRU = total fructose | GLU = total glucose („dextrose") | SOR = sorbitol | SUC = sucrose, „sugar"

☺ well tolerated | ☹ not tolerated | ☺ sometimes tolerated – individual testing during the test phase recommended

FOOD / PRODUCT	ED	PD	FREE FRU	FREE GLU	FREE SUC	FRU	GLU	GLU/ FRU
apple	☹	☹	5.9	2.4	2.1	6.9	3.4	0.5
apricot	☹	☺	0.9	1.7	5.1	3.4	4.3	1.3
artichoke	😐	☺	1.7	0.8				0.4
asparagus	😐	☺	0.9	0.8	0.3	1.1	0.9	0.8
avocado	☺	☺	0.2	0.1	0.1	0.3	0.2	0.6
bamboo shoots	😐	☺	0.4	0.4	0.2	0.5	0.5	0.9
banana	😐	😐	3.4	3.6				1.0
beef *	☺	☺	-	-	-	-	-	-
beer (lager) *	☹	😐	-	-	-	-	-	-
beetroot	😐	😐	0.3	0.3	7.9	4.2	4.2	1.0
blackberry	😐	😐	3.1	3.0		3.1	3.0	1.0
blueberry	😐	☺	3.4	2.5		3.4	2.5	0.7
brie cheese	☺	☺	0.0	0.0	0.0	0.0	0.0	
broccoli	😐	☺	1.1	1.1	0.5	1.4	1.3	1.0
brown ale*	☹	☹	-	-	-	-	-	-
brussels sprouts	😐	😐	0.8	0.9				1.1
buttermilk	☺	☺						
cabbage	☹	😐	1.8	2.0				1.2
camel milk	☺	☺						
camembert cheese	☺	☺						
canned tuna *	😐	☺	-	-	-	-	-	-
carrot	😐	☺	1.3	1.4	2.1	2.4	2.5	1.0
cauliflower	😐	😐	0.9	1.0		0.9	1.0	1.1
celeriac	😐	☺	0.1	0.0				0.0
cep	😐	☺	0.3	0.3				1.0
champagne *	☹	😐	-	-	-	-	-	-
chanterelle	😐	☺	0.1	0.1				1.4
chard	☺	☺	0.3	0.2	0.2	0.4	0.3	0.8
cheddar cheese	☺	☺	0.0	0.0	0.0	0.0	0.0	
cherry	☹	☹	6.0	7.0				1.2
chestnuts	😐	😐	0.0	0.0	11.3	5.7	5.7	1.0
chickpea	😐	😐	0.1	0.1				1.0
chicken *	☺	☺	-	-	-	-	-	-
chicory	☺	☺	0.7	1.3	0.5	0.9	1.5	1.6

FOOD / PRODUCT	ED	PD	FREE FRU	FREE GLU	FREE SUC	FRU	GLU	GLU/ FRU
chinese cabbage	☺	☺	0.5	0.7	0.0	0.5	0.7	1.3
cocoa powder	☺	☺	0.0	0.0	2.2	1.1	1.1	1.0
coconut	☺	☺	0.0	0.2	4.6	2.3	2.5	1.1
coconut milk	☺	☺	0.0	0.2	3.0	1.5	1.7	1.1
cod	☺	☺	0.0	0.0	0.0	0.0	0.0	
coffee	☺	☺						
corn (canned)	☺	☺	0.4	0.6	2.2	1.5	1.7	1.1
corn (fresh)	☺	☺	0.4	0.6	2.2	1.5	1.7	1.1
cottage cheese *	☺	☺	-	-	-	-	-	-
courgette (see zucchini)								
cream 10% fat	☹	☺	0.0	0.0	0.1	0.0	0.0	1.0
cucumber	☺	☺	0.9	0.9		0.9	0.9	1.0
currant	☺	☺	3.0	3.0				1.0
dandelion leaves	☺	☺	0.6	1.3	0.5	0.8	1.5	1.9
diet soda	☺	☺	0.0	0.0		0.0	0.0	
dried date	☹	☹	24.9	25.0				1.0
dried fig	☹	☹	23.5	25.7	5.9	26.5	28.7	1.1
edam cheese	☺	☺	0.0	0.0	0.0	0.0	0.0	
egg	☺	☺	0.0	0.4				
eggplant	☺	☺	1.0	1.0				1.0
emmentaler cheese *	☺	☺	0.0	0.0	0.0	0.0	0.0	
energy drink, diet *	☹	☹	0.0	0.0	-	0.0	0.0	-
energy drink *	☹	☹	-	-	-	-	-	-
fennel	☺	☺	1.1	1.3				1.2
fig	☹	☺	5.6	7.0	0.5	5.9	7.2	1.2
fish. fresh or frozen *	☺	☺	-	-	-	-	-	-
garlic	☺	☺	3.2	2.1	3.3	4.9	3.8	0.8
goat cheese *	☺	☺	-	-	-	-	-	-
goat's milk	☺	☺	0.0	0.0	0.0	0.0	0.0	
gooseberry	☹	☺	3.3	3.0				0.9
grain (wheat grain)	☺	☺	0.0					0.0
grapefruit	☺	☺	2.1	2.4	3.0	3.6	3.9	1.1
grapes	☹	☹	7.4	7.2				1.0
green beans	☺	☺	1.3	1.0		1.3	1.0	0.7

FOOD / PRODUCT	ED	PD	FREE FRU	FREE GLU	FREE SUC	FRU	GLU	GLU/ FRU
ham. raw or cooked ☺	☺	-	-	-	-	-	-	-
herring	☺	☺	0.0	0.0	0.0	0.0	0.0	
honey	☹	☹	38.8	33.9		38.8	33.9	0.9
horseradish	☺	☺	0.1	1.4	6.7	3.5	4.8	1.4
kaki	☹	☺	8.0	7.0				0.9
kale	☺	☺	0.9	0.6		0.9	0.6	0.7
kiwi	☹	☺	4.6	4.3	0.2	4.7	4.4	0.9
kohlrabi TURNIP	☺	☺	1.2	1.4				1.1
lamb's lettuce	☺	☺	0.2	0.4	0.2	0.3	0.5	1.5
leek (allium)	☹	☺	1.2	1.0	0.8	1.7	1.4	0.9
lemon	☺	☺	0.9	1.0	0.6	1.2	1.3	1.1
lima bean	☹	☺	0.5	0.1				0.1
lime	☺	☺	0.8	0.8				1.0
liver. beef *	☺	☺	-	-	-	-	-	-
low-fat milk	☺	☺						
lychee	☺	☺	3.2	5.0				1.6
malt *	☹	☹	-	-	-	-	-	-
mandarin. tangerine	☺	☺	1.3	1.7	7.1	4.8	5.2	1.1
mango	☹	☹	2.6	0.9	9.5	7.4	5.6	0.8
mare's milk *	☺	☺	-	-	-	-	-	-
mozzarella	☺	☺						
mushrooms	☺	☺	0.2	0.2		0.2	0.2	1.0
musk melon	☺	☺						
natural yoghurt 3.5%	☺	☺						
okra	☺	☺	0.8	0.6	0.6	1.1	0.9	0.8
onion	☹	☺	1.3	1.6				1.2
orange	☹	☺	2.5	2.2				0.9
papaya	☺	☺	0.3	1.0				3.0
parmesan cheese	☺	☺						
parsley leaf	☺	☺	0.3	0.5				1.7
parsley root	☺	☺	0.7	0.6				0.8
parsnip	☺	☺	0.3	0.2	2.6	1.5	1.5	1.0
peach	☹	☺	1.2	1.0		1.2	1.0	0.8
pear	☹	☹	6.7	1.7		6.7	1.7	0.2

131

FOOD / PRODUCT	ED	PD	FREE FRU	FREE GLU	FREE SUC	FRU	GLU	GLU/ FRU
peas	☺	☺	0.1	0.1				1.4
pepper (green)	☺	☺	1.3	1.4				1.1
pickles *	☺	☺	-	-	-	-	-	-
pineapple	☹	☹	2.1	1.7	6.0	5.1	4.7	0.9
plum	☹	☹	2.0	3.4		2.0	3.4	1.7
pomegranate	☹	☺	7.9	7.2		7.9	7.2	0.9
pork *	☺	☺	-	-	-	-	-	-
potato	☺	☺	0.2	0.2	0.3	0.3	0.4	1.2
prickly pear	☺	☺	0.6	6.5				10.8
pumpkin (hokkaido)	☺	☺	1.3	1.5		1.3	1.5	1.1
radishes	☺	☺	0.7	1.3	0.1	0.8	1.4	1.7
raisin	☹	☹	31.6	31.2				1.0
raspberry	☺	☺	2.1	1.8		2.1	1.8	0.9
red cabbage	☺	☺	1.3	1.7		1.3	1.7	1.3
red wine *	☹	☺	-	-	-	-	-	-
rhubarb	☺	☺	0.4	0.4				1.0
rice	☺	☺	0.0	0.0	0.2	0.1	0.1	1.0
roquefort	☺	☺						
salad (green. lettuce)	☺	☺	0.5	0.5	0.1	0.6	0.5	0.9
salami *	☺	☺	-	-	-	-	-	-
salmon	☺	☺	0.0	0.0	0.0	0.0	0.0	
salsify	☺	☺	0.1	0.0				0.2
sauerkraut *	☹	☹	0.2	0.4				2.0
schnaps	☹	☺						
sheep's cheese	☺	☺						
sheep's milk	☺	☺	0.0	0.0	0.0	0.0	0.0	
skimmed milk	☺	☺						
skimmed milk powder*	☺	☺	-	-	-	-	-	-
sour cream	☺	☺	0.0	0.0	0.0	0.0	0.0	
soybean	☺	☺		0.0	5.7	2.8	2.8	1.0
spinach	☺	☺	0.1	0.1	0.2	0.2	0.2	1.1
sprouts, fresh	☺	☺	-	-	-	-	-	-
strawberry	☹	☺	2.3	2.2				0.9
sweet potato	☺	☺	0.7	0.8	3.2	2.3	2.4	1.1

FOOD / PRODUCT	ED	PD	FREE FRU	FREE GLU	FREE SUC	FRU	GLU	GLU/ FRU
sweet whey	☺	☺	0.0	0.0	0.0	0.0	0.0	
tangerine (see mandarin)								
tomato	☹	☺	1.4	1.1				0.8
turkey *	☺	☺	-	-	-	-	-	-
turnip (see kohlrabi)								
watermelon	☺	☺	3.9	2.0				0.5
wheat beer *	☹	☹	-	-	-	-	-	-
whey powder *	☺	☺	-	-	-	-	-	-
white wine *	☹	☺	-	-	-	-	-	-
whole milk	☺	☺	0.0			0.0		
whole milk powder	☺	☺	0.0	0.0	0.0	0.0	0.0	
yeast extract *	☺	☺	-	-	-	-	-	-
yeast	☺	☺				0.0	0.0	
zucchini	☺	☺	1.1	1.0				0.9

* No value can be assigned for various reasons. The product, for example, exists in many varieties with different levels of sugars

Histamine list alphabetically sorted

ED = elimination diet | PD = permanent diet
☺ well tolerated | 😐 sometimes tolerated – individual testing during the test phase recommended | ☹ poorly tolerated

Food	ED	PD	Food	ED	PD
Apple	😐	☺	Lamb's lettuce	☺	☺
Apricot	😐	☺	Leek	😐	☺
Artichoke	😐	☺	Lemons	☹	😐
Asparagus	☺	☺	Lettuce	☺	☺
Aubergine	☹	😐	Lima beans	☹	😐
Avocado	☹	😐	Limes	☹	😐
Bamboo shoots	☹	😐	Lychee	😐	☺
Banana	☹	😐	Malt beer	☹	😐
Beef	☺	☺	Mandarin / Tangerine	☹	😐
Beer	☹	☹	Mango	😐	☺
Beetroot	😐	☺	Mangold	😐	😐
Bell peppers (green)	☹	😐	Mushrooms	☹	😐
Black salsify	😐	☺	Okra	😐	☺
Blackberry	😐	☺	Onions	😐	😐
Blueberries	☺	☺	Orange	☹	☹
Broccoli	☺	☺	Papaya	😐	😐
Brussels sprouts	😐	😐	Parsnip	😐	😐
Carrots	☺	☺	Peach	😐	☺
Cauliflower	😐	☺	Pears	☹	😐
Celeriac	😐	😐	Peas	☹	😐

Food	ED	PD	Food	ED	PD
Chanterelle mushrooms	☹	☺	Pickled cucumber	☹	☹
Cherry	☺	☺	Pineapple	☹	☹
Chicken (without skin)	☺	☺	Plums	☹	☺
Chickpeas	☹	☺	Pomegranate	☺	☺
Chicory	☺	☺	Porcini (Ceps)	☹	☺
Chinese cabbage	☺	☺	Pork	☺	☺
Cocoa powder	☹	☺	Potato	☹	☺
Coconut milk	☺	☺	Prickly pear	☺	☺
Coffee	☺	☺	Pumpkin (Hokkaido)	☺	☺
Corn (tinned)	☹	☺	Radish	☺	☺
Corn, fresh, cooked	☺	☺	Raisins	☹	☺
Courgettes / Zucchini	☺	☺	Raspberries	☺	☺
Cucumber	☺	☺	Red cabbage	☹	☺
Dandelion leaves	☺	☺	Redcurrents	☺	☺
Dates, dried	☹	☺	Rhubarb	☺	☺
Egg	☺	☺	Rice	☹	☺
Endive	☺	☺	Sauerkraut	☹	☹
Energy drink with sugar	☹	☹	Savoy cabbage	☹	☺
Energy drink, sugar-free	☹	☹	Sodas, diet	☹	☺
Fennel	☺	☺	Soy beans	☹	☺
Figs	☹	☺	Spinach	☹	☺
Figs, dried	☹	☺	Spirits, distilled	☹	☺
fish, fresh water	☺	☺	Strawberries	☹	☹
fish, salt water (no tuna!)	☺	☺	Sugar melon	☹	☺
Fruit teas, fresh brewed	☺	☺	Sweet chestnuts	☺	☺

135

Food	ED	PD	Food	ED	PD
Garlic	☹	😐	Sweet potatoes	☺	☺
Gooseberry	😐	☺	Tangerine / Mandarin	☹	😐
Grapefruit	☹	☹	Tomato	☹	☹
Grapes	😐	😐	Tuna, fresh	☹	😐
Green beans	☹	😐	Tuna, tinned	☹	☹
Honey	😐	☺	Watermelon	☺	☺
Hoseraddish	☹	😐	Wheat beer	☹	☹
Kaki	😐	☺	White cabbage	☹	😐
Kiwi	☹	☹	Wine, red	☹	☹
Kohlrabi	😐	☺	Wine, white	☹	☹

Links that might help you

www.food-intolerance-network.com

The food intolerance network (fin) is a charity that provides information about lactose intolerance, fructose intolerance, histamine intolerance and most other food intolerances.

fin on Facebook   facebook.com/foodintolerance

fin on Pinterest   pinterest.com/foodintolerance

www.histamineintolerance.org.uk

Website by Genny Masterman with information on histamine intolerance.

http://www.allergyuk.org/

UK's leading medical charity dealing with allergy

http://www.fda.gov/

US Food and Drug Administration (FDA)

Dietetic Associations

British Dietetic Association   http://www.bda.uk.com/

American Dietetic Association   http://www.eatright.org/

Dieticians of Canada   http://www.dietitians.ca/

Dietitians Association of Australia   http://www.daa.asn.au/

20924546R00080

Made in the USA
Middletown, DE
12 June 2015